Manhood

Manhood

The Rise and Fall of the Penis

Mels van Driel

REAKTION BOOKS

Published by Reaktion Books Ltd
33 Great Sutton Street
London EC1V 0DX, UK
www.reaktionbooks.co.uk

The original edition of this book was first published in 2008
bv Uitgeverij De Arbeiderspers, Amsterdam, under the title
Geheime delen: Alles wat je er altijd al over wilde weten
© Mels van Driel and Arbeiderspers 2008

English-language translation © Reaktion Books Ltd 2009

English translation by Paul Vincent

This publication has been made possible
with financial support from the
Foundation for the Production and Translation of Dutch Literature.

Printed and bound in Great Britain
by Cromwell Press Group, Trowbridge, Wiltshire

British Library Cataloguing in Publication Data
Driel, Mels van, 1954–
    Manhood : the rise and fall of the penis.
    1. Penis. 2. Men–Sexual behavior.
    1. Title
    612.6'1–dc22

ISBN: 978 1 86189 542 4

Contents

Introduction

Everyone knows what it's like to become hooked on a particular subject. These things never happen purely by chance; in all probability they relate to something in us. We are drawn to the topic as if by a magnet. It can reach the point where the person concerned is obsessed day and night. There is a constant stream of new facts, ideas and insights. Of course you're now probably thinking that the writer himself has, or had, fertility problems or some erectile dysfunction. Well, that isn't the case, but that doesn't mean it won't be at some point in the future. The same is true of all my male readers.

My broad interest derives mainly from daily contact with men's 'private parts'. Since mid-1983 I have worked as a urologist, so that I deal more or less permanently with sick people, or with people who think they're sick. In the last few decades tens of thousands of penises and testicles have been through my hands. Eventually one feels the urge to dig deeper. Why do men come to doctors complaining about these organs?

Over the years my thinking about men's 'family jewels' has achieved a precarious balance between urological, sexological and psychological perspectives, the academic approach, the problems of my surgery, daily life and especially literature. This is what moved me to write this book.

Wearing several different hats as a writer isn't necessarily always easy, but it does provide a broad, human perspective, through a kind of internal cross-fertilization. Of course novels and poetry have the last word; art always takes precedence over science. But for a urologist the fact that the testicles and the penis are also organs, which if necessary must go under the knife, is in itself a source of satisfaction!

Drop the word castration in mixed company and watch all the men grab for their crotch, rather like footballers in a wall protecting themselves from a direct free kick. This reflex can in fact be traced back to the ideas of Sigmund Freud (1856–1939). Having been circumcised, like most Jews and Muslims, he used the term 'castration' to denote the removal of the penis, though over the centuries castration has never meant anything anywhere in the world but the removal of the testicles. Freud's successful coup is particularly interesting because in his thinking the testicles had lost all significance: he shifted almost all the focus onto the penis and the symbolic phallus, although the root of fertility and virility lies elsewhere, namely in the testicles. That shift was prompted by another: from sex as a means of procreation to sex for pleasure. In the wake of this development, increasing attention was paid to the penis at the expense of the testicles. This book attempts to redress the balance. The testicles receive at least as much attention as the penis, while the prostate and the seminal vesicles, also important in reproduction, are also briefly discussed.

In this book the genitalia are linked to such phenomena as religion, death and our craving for sexual pleasure. It describes how people down the ages have thought about the male private parts, and have had themselves castrated and sterilized. In addition it lists genital ailments, some serious, some not, and the relevant treatments. In addition a great number of secrets are uncovered. This information is interspersed with the thoughts and experiences of celebrities, poets and novelists. I lay absolutely no claim to completeness or scholarly rigour.

Not all readers will be aware that the Bible contains everything that life has to offer in terms of sex and love. It includes, for example (in alphabetical order): abortion, adultery, aphrodisiacs, anal sex, bestiality, castration, circumcision, exhibitionism, gang rape, group sex, homosexuality, oppression of women, phallus worship, partner-swapping, prostitution, Satanic sex, sex during menstruation, sexually transmitted diseases and, of course, self-abuse. This makes it impossible not to include a number of stories from various books in the Bible.

The best novels and poems commonly mirror everyday reality. One needs only the slightest familiarity with literary history to know that many writers have celebrated the healthy human body as a rich source of happiness and pleasure. There are, though, also writers, poets and philosophers who have written extremely graphically and evocatively about balls, penises and prostates or about ailments of those organs – often in a way that no expert could improve on. Writers and poets, major and minor, male and female, undoubtedly have a broader, more human view of reality. Some female poets eagerly explore the scrotum, while the willy and the balls are mocked with great relish. Sometimes the private parts are dangerous and sometimes a set of toys. It is not only writers and poets who provide knowledge and ideas; the same is true of singers, both castrati and others. A long series of interviews, conducted over 25 years with men suffering from major and minor ailments of the genitalia, guarantees a high level of authenticity. Several of these have been included with names deleted as short 'case histories'.

Who is this book aimed at? Principally, certainly, at the 'worried well', with their fretting about pain, reduced fertility, erectile dysfunction, unusual swellings, undescended testicles, prostate cancer, castration anxiety and so on and so on. It offers women the opportunity of gaining a better understanding of their men. Men and women contemplating sterilization will find this book particularly useful. It offers arguments on who should and should not 'go through with it'.

Its diversity of content makes the book resemble a big bag of liquorice allsorts. And as with liquorice allsorts, it's best not to eat everything in one go. I have kept the tone light – the most effective way to approach ditherers and fretters.

chapter one

The Testicles and the Scrotum

Terminology

Ancient Greek and Latin had a great variety of terms for the testicles. Only a few of these have remained in use. Some years ago two Classical scholars, Horstmanhoff and Beukers, devoted a study to the subject. The Greek word for ball is *orchis*, which is found, for instance, in medical parlance. An 'orchidectomy' is an operation for the removal of the testicles, while an inflammation of a testicle as a result of mumps is known in the jargon as *mumps orchitis*. Orchids are so called because the tubers of the flower show some similarity to testicles. In the Middle Ages it was thought that the man who ate the biggest of these tubers would sire especially large children.

Testis means witness in Latin, as evidenced by such words as 'testify' and 'testament', a document drawn up by a lawyer and signed in the presence of witnesses. The Dutch expression 'the lawyer and the witnesses' for the penis and the testicles recalls this link, as does the phrase 'the lawyer inside and the witnesses outside' describing sexual intercourse with the penis in the vagina and the balls dangling outside. (Don't assume that this can be taken for granted: a form of coitus exists in which both penis and balls are inserted in the vagina.)

All kinds of factors may give words that were originally neutral in meaning enhanced or diminished status, moving from obscene to scientific or alternatively from respectably descriptive to coarse. The Anglo-Saxon 'bollocks', for example, was for centuries a purely descriptive term (see its use in the medieval translation of *Reynard the Fox* below), but today is considered vulgar. It refers to the testicles, literally and figuratively, in widespread uses like 'Bollocks!' (nonsense), or 'He thinks he's the dog's bollocks' (He has an unduly high opinion of himself). Neither of these expressions is current in the USA.

'Ball-bag' and 'nut-sack' are current slang for 'scrotum', though they have not yet ousted the technical term in everyday usage. 'Having balls' is synonymous with having backbone and can be extended to resolute women like ex-premier Margaret Thatcher. Other informal words for testicles include crown jewels, goolies, nads and nadgers. In this book 'testicles', 'testes' and 'balls' are used indiscriminately.

Scrotum remains the standard medical term for the bag of skin containing the testicles. The word is a medieval form of *scortum*, hide or skin, which in Latin may have referred to a leather quiver. The concept of a scrotal 'pouch', less crude than 'sack' or 'bag', has a long history. The image is found, for example, in the medieval Dutch poem of *Reynard the Fox*, where Tibert the cat, venting his anger on a village priest, bites off the priest's 'stitchless satchel/with which a man rings the bell' (in the translation of A. J. Barnouw and E. College). This castration scene contains a number of other euphemisms, including 'thing', 'innards' and a little later 'bells'. In one version of the poem, that used by William Caxton for his 1481 translation, it is clear that the castration is in fact only partial: the priest loses, we are told, 'his right cullion or ballock stone'. The use of the ecclesiastic image of bells is noteworthy. In Sylvia Hubers' contemporary poem 'Of Course!' the bells make a challenging comeback:

> Of course!
> I've got rat-arsed again.
> Of course
> Can't put one foot in front of the other
> anymore.
> But it's too late now
> for kiddies' games.
> Come on now, it's your turn
> to show me some of that
> bell-ringing
> you've spent all evening
> bragging about!!

In the same way that 'bag' or 'sack' are not particularly kind terms for scrotum, but are common, the same is true of 'ball' for testicle. To turn to failing virility for a moment: 'brewer's droop' is temporary, alcohol-induced impotence, while being 'out of gas' may describe a more permanent condition.

Greek and Latin had a plethora of words for penis, only a few of which are still current. It is often difficult to determine why one word has survived and another has not. Most are metaphors, and the most obvious references are to length, cylindrical form and vertical position. Sometimes the image was of the stalk of a plant, the shaft of a spear or the blade of a sword, sometimes the upright warp of a woven fabric (*stêma* in Greek) or the bronze-plated, wedge-shaped ship's nose (*embolon*) with which vessels tried to ram each other in ancient sea battles. The usual anatomical name for the female sexual organ, 'vagina' (sheath), is a perfect complement to the blade of the sword, while the term 'ejaculation' relates to Latin *iaculum* (a small spear). So that an *eiaculatio* is the hurling of one's seed, like a spear. Ample imagery to choose from. The choice eventually fell on 'penis', though the precise origin remains vague. Some philologists see it as deriving from the Latin verb *pendere* (hang, droop), which might be seen as appropriate in some cases.

Penis, then, has made it big. Any English-speaker wanting to avoid four-letter words and graphic Anglo-Saxon terms will undoubtedly resort to this scientific designation. The previously mentioned Classicists Horstmanshoff and Beukers regard the now archaic *man's yard*, like Dutch *roede* (rod), German *Ruthe* and French *verge*, as loan translations of the Arabic *al-kamarah*, a term used in antiquity in the influential Arab medical literature. Via Latin *virga* (twig, branch) the image was adopted by Western European languages.

Sanskrit on the other hand uses completely different metaphors for the male member, while Sheikh Nefzawi's *Perfumed Garden* mentions, for example:

the dove, because the moment it begins to flag, the stiff penis resembles a dove brooding its eggs.

the tinkler, because every time it enters and leaves the vagina, the member makes a sound.

the untamable one, because as soon as it is erect it starts to move and does not stop till it has found the entrance to the vulva, which it then shamelessly penetrates without so much as a by-your-leave.

the liberator, since by penetrating the vulva of a woman who has been thrice rejected, it gives this woman the freedom to return to her first husband.

the rod, since the member inches slowly up the woman's thighs towards her *mons Veneris* and creeps inside, until it has nestled there to its satisfaction and achieves an ejaculation.

the crowbar, since if access to the vulva is difficult, the member as it were forces its way in, breaking and trampling everything in its path, like a wild animal on heat.

the bald one, since the member is hairless!

In the Middle Ages, according to the Dutch writer Hans van Straten, the penis was called the *caulis*, or stalk, referring to its rigid state. A host of designations from Shakespearean times and later include: thing, anchovy, tree of life, shuttle, manhood, artillery, baldpate friar, glister syringe, devil, pintle, yard, jiggumbob, monkey's tail, bodkin, pego, chitterling, whim-wham, shaft, date, key, robin, bilbo, sceptre, flute, nutcracker, date, maypole, spoon, thorn, wand, mast, quill, touch-finger, sword, tarriwang and crest. The wealth of contemporary terms is easily accessible online.

Fertilization

For many centuries notions of human reproduction were based on the ideas formulated long before the beginning of the first millennium by two Greek authorities, Hippocrates (460–377 BC) and Aristotle (380–322 BC). In his book *De Semine* (On Semen) the former wrote that both male and female seminal fluid was formed in the brain and subsequently reached the genitalia via the spine. When both substances united in sexual intercourse, this would produce a child that would inherit the characteristics of either the father or the mother, depending on which of the seminal fluids provided by the father and mother was more powerful. According to Hippocrates the sex of the child was also determined by the strength of the seminal fluid.

While Hippocrates assigned a more or less equal role to the man and the woman, Aristotle took a different view. Of course he could not help admitting some female input and so argued that woman's sole contribution was to provide what he called *catamenia*. This was residual menstrual blood that constituted transformed matter and could basically produce nothing until the man added his seed. The drawings of Leonardo da Vinci (1452–1519) show his brilliant mind still clinging to the idea that seminal fluid came straight from the brain. Leonardo drew two ducts in the penis, one for the passage of urine and one for seminal fluid. The white seminal fluid came like mother's milk directly from the backbone. Leonardo was interested not only in helicopters, but also in reproduction. In the Royal Gallery at Windsor there is a cross-section drawn by him of a man and woman having intercourse. Above the sketch he wrote, in his familiar mirror writing: 'I show people the first, or perhaps second reason for their existence.' For his anatomical drawings he used animals such as oxen as a model. This led him astray: he forgot to draw the prostate, which is understandable, since in the case of castration before puberty that organ develops scarcely if at all. Even a genius like Leonardo, then, got it wrong not once, but twice.

One of the many researchers who tackled the mystery of procreation was William Harvey (1578–1657), the discoverer of the circulation of the blood. After his appointment as Physician Extraordinary to King James I he concentrated his research on the growth of the embryo in chickens' eggs and on the uteri of deer from the Royal Deer Park. In 1651, at the age of 73, he published his research findings. In contrast to the views then current, Harvey asserted that animals and human beings came from an egg, with the exception of insects, which, he maintained, were generated 'spontaneously' from waste matter. The latter was Aristotle's ancient notion, to which Harvey adhered in another respect too: he ascribed the development of the embryo to the vital forces in the male sperm.

Aristotle's ideas on spontaneous generation in insects and other invertebrates were made less plausible by the investigations of a physician at the court of Tuscany, Francesco Redi (1626–1697), which demonstrated that flies lay eggs in meat waste. The starting point for his studies was a passage of Classical poetry. In Book XIX of Homer's *Iliad*, Achilles is worried that the flies in the wounds of his slain friend Patroclus will produce worms. Redi examined exactly what Homer meant and observed that after a while worms (i.e. maggots) emerged from meat on which flies had settled. No worms appeared where insects had no access. He used an amazing range of different meats: ox, venison, buffalo, lion, tiger, dog, lamb, kid, rabbit, duck, goose, chicken, swallow, swordfish, tuna, eel, tongue, etc. The result was always the same, and he drew the conclusion that insects were not produced by rotting waste matter, but also came from eggs, which the mother laid in the meat for nutriment.

The celebrated anatomist Frederik Ruysch (1638–1731) was equally sceptical that fertilization could take place 'solely through the vapours and spirits of the male seed'. 'I am well aware that in sexual congress the larger part of the seed flows away, but I am convinced that the viscous seed remaining in the womb is sufficient to bring about fertilization.' Ruysch had found the uterine cavity and the two 'trumpets' (Fallopian tubes) filled with a very large quantity of male seed. This was most unusual: Harvey had never been able to find seed in the uteri of deer, but Ruysch *had* found it in women. (In the 1970s Harvey's findings were examined in the light of modern knowledge by Professor Roger Short, who also made a remarkable film replicating Harvey's research. In hindsight it was no wonder that Harvey did not discover how reproduction actually functioned, mainly because this is much less transparent in deer than in most other animals. And of course without a microscope it was very difficult for him to detect sperm in the uteri of the hinds he dissected shortly after mating.)

One day Ruysch had a unique opportunity. He was commissioned by the Amsterdam municipal authorities to write a report on a murder. The victim was a prostitute, whose throat had been cut by a young man with whom she had just had intercourse. After establishing the cause of death, Ruysch satisfied his scientific curiosity, with three doctors in attendance. He cut open the victim's abdomen, 'being most curious to see what would appear in the womb and those parts made for conception. I therefore removed the womb, the Fallopian tubes and their appendages very carefully from the body,' he noted. The cervix was closed, but when he pressed gently with his finger it opened and sperm came out. He then opened the womb and found more sperm. Both tubes were also full of it. He preserved the material in his 'balsamic' fluid, which caused the sperm to harden and stabilize. Subsequently it could serve as scientific evidence.

Later Ruysch had a further opportunity to gather first-hand evidence. This time it involved the body of a wife caught in the act with her lover and stabbed to death by her husband. Ruysch was called in to perform a post-mortem examination, and when he found the womb somewhat more 'elevated' than normal, he suspected that fertilization had taken place. He then removed the womb from the body for further examination, and found her lover's sperm not only in the uterine cavity, but also in both Fallopian tubes.

Ruysch's assumption was that if the seed itself were not necessary to effect fertilization, the tubes would not be full of sperm. When asked, most women had told him that when they became pregnant they usually had the feeling that most of the sperm had remained in their bodies. 'What else is one to believe than that the substances of nature, and not only their vapours or spirits are required for this work,' observed Ruysch. The question of whether the sperm contained tiny creatures, which also played a part, he left unresolved.

For centuries Aristotle's view on the predominant role of the male in reproduction obviously had a great appeal for many people, including another scientist, Antonie van Leeuwenhoek (1632–1723). Using candlelight and ground glass he had made his own microscope. He was actually a cloth merchant by trade and also ran a draper's shop, where he sold buttons and ribbons. In the back room behind the shop he became a self-trained scientist. He taught himself glass-blowing, grinding and polishing and was subsequently able to produce high-quality lenses. During his lifetime he ground over five hundred, including some with a magnification of approximately 480x. No one knows why Van Leeuwenhoek started using the microscope. Perhaps he wanted to take a close look at textiles, or he may have simply revelled in his own ingenuity and skill. His simple microscope was not much more than a wooden frame containing a small glass globe, made by extending a thin length of red-hot glass until a globule separated from it which after cooling was polished smooth. It was certainly not easy to use the apparatus. Endless peering, from very close range, and preferably in bright sunlight, soon led to tired eyes. Van Leeuwenhoek had an additional problem: he could not draw at all. For this reason he employed a number of draughtsmen, who made illustrations for him.

A Leiden professor was very interested in the cloth merchant's work. He introduced a relative of his, the student Johan Ham, to Van Leeuwenhoek. On his second visit, in 1677, Ham brought with him the sperm of a man with the clap. He had seen tiny creatures moving about in it and assumed that their presence was connected with the man's disease. He asked Van Leeuwenhoek to take a look with his microscope. A few years before, at the request of a foreign scholar, Van Leeuwenhoek had put spittle, sweat and sperm under his microscope and at that time had seen something resembling tiny globules in the sperm, but had not pursued his observations because he found them distasteful. Now he was urged by the student to repeat the investigation. Van Leeuwenhoek felt extremely uncomfortable. The reason was that in his follow-up studies he used his own sperm and to avoid accusations of sinful behaviour felt obliged to explain that the observations had been carried out on sperm left over after sexual relations with his wife Cornelia. On another occasion he reported that he had placed the sperm under the microscope within ten seconds of ejaculation. His research showed that the creatures Johan Ham had seen were also found in fresh, healthy sperm. He called them spermatozoa. On the basis of ancient metaphysical writings he thought initially that he saw portions of microscopic homunculi, tiny male creatures swimming about in the seminal fluid. On 3 December 1677, not feeling entirely sure of himself, he wrote to the Royal Society in London: 'If your Harvey and our De Graaf had seen a hundredth part of what I have seen, they would have agreed with my finding that the man's seed forms the embryo by itself, and all the woman can contribute is to receive or nourish the male seed.' And in so doing he in fact confirmed what the Greek playwright Aeschylus (525–456 BC) had written many centuries before: 'The mother of what is called her child, is not its parent, but only the nurse of the young life sown in her.'

Van Leeuwenhoek lived to be ninety and continued with microscopic research until his death in August 1723, fifty years after his introduction to the Royal Society by Reinier de Graaf (1641–1673). His daughter sent his collection of microscopes and specimens to London, where it eventually disappeared, so that only a few of his better microscopes survive in museums, where visitors are usually more interested in the silver slides and the adjustment knob than in the most important component: the tiny glass globule that served as a lens. With his microscopes Van Leeuwenhoek had found the answer to the problem Harvey and Reinier de Graaf had wrestled with: semen played a direct physical role in reproduction, the reason being that spermatozoa could find their way to the womb. He had dismissed the views deriving from, for instance, the work of Redi, Jan Swammerdam (1637–1680) and De Graaf, in which the ovum played a central role in reproduction. Van Leeuwenhoek had focused on the male aspect, while the others had had looked mainly at the female side.

The argument on the question as to what was more important: the ovum or the spermatozoon, between ovists and animaculists (also called *spermists*) was not finally decided until the second half of the nineteenth century, in 1875 to be exact. In that year the German anatomist Wilhelm Hertwig (1849–1922) showed in an animal experiment that fertilization comes about through the merging of the nuclei of the ovum and the spermatozoon. The exact process was revealed only in 1944, when John Rock of Harvard University put a human ovum in a dish and added a drop of living human sperm. After placing this mixture in human blood serum, Rock was the first person to observe the division of the fertilized ovum into two, the beginning of a strange process that some nine months later results in the birth of a new human being.

Today we know that the female ovum contains more than half the information necessary for the future human being. It provides not only 23 nuclear chromosomes to complement the 23 from the spermatozoon, but also the cytoplasmatic DNA located in the mitochondria, the genes of which derive exclusively from the mother. The mitochondria are simply tiny power stations in the cell. This fact torpedoes the arrogant notion that the father is most important in reproduction. More of that anon!

Hanging left

As regards appearance there is great diversity in the protuberances we have given the prosaic name of scrotum. Scrotums may be large or small, long or short, smooth or wrinkled, heavily or lightly pigmented, nicely rounded or extremely asymmetrical. In fourteenth-century Europe high-ranking nobles were allowed to walk around with naked genitals under their short tunics. Their tight-fitting short breeches were not closed at the crotch. If their private parts were not sufficiently large to dangle about alluringly, they wore a *braquette*, a set of simulated genitalia in leather. Later, in the fifteenth and sixteenth centuries, another ornament came into fashion, the so-called codpiece (*cod* means scrotum), which was sometimes embroidered or encrusted with jewels. It was a final relic of the age of chivalry, and today's double-stitched fly may be the last of the codpiece.

The left testicle usually hangs slightly lower than the right. This has nothing to do with being left- or right-handed. The anomaly is probably due to the fact that in most men the left testicle is slightly larger and heavier than the right. As a result the penis also usually 'hangs left', as the saying goes.

Until quite recently tailors making a bespoke suit asked their customer whether he 'dressed left or right', so that extra material could be sewn in to camouflage as far as possible the effect of dribbling after urination. The modern clothing industry certainly also takes this into account: the better makes of menswear cut the front of the left leg of a pair of trousers three-quarters of a centimetre wider as standard!

Apart from that, opinions differ on whether the scrotum couldn't have been made slightly more appealing in appearance and on whether the positioning of the scrotum couldn't have been a little more convenient, certainly in an age when cycle sports are exceptionally popular. After all, in many animals the semen-producing organs are tucked neatly into the abdominal cavity. In rodents and prosimians, for example, the testicles descend only in the mating season and subsequently return to the abdomen. This is not the case in man or in his oldest domesticated animals. Recent research has shown that the positioning of the testicles is mainly connected with the lifestyle of the species. This actually undermines the 'balls-as-coolbox' theory (of which more below). Animals that move fluidly have their sperm-factories enclosed in their bodies, while those that run, jump, jolt and bump, were better off with testicles located externally.

Long before birth the testicles and epididymides are formed in a place at the back of and high above the abdominal cavity, in the vicinity of the kidneys. From there the testicles descend down a kind of slide formed by the back of the bulging abdominal membrane, towards the inguinal canal at the bottom of the abdomen. If everything goes to plan in the last three months of pregnancy the testicles and accompanying seminal ducts and blood vessels descend through that inguinal canal into the scrotum. The above explanation is not totally accurate, since in fact the testicles gradually move lower and lower as the body grows lengthways. Be that as it may, in approximately 95 per cent of 'full-term' males the testicles are in the appointed place around the time of birth. It may happen that the testicles remain within the abdomen. When this occurs in a male pig the animal is known as a 'cryptorchid boar' or sometimes, more colloquially, a 'rig pig'.

A true cryptorchid boar takes at least ten minutes to complete ejaculation of his sperm – two coffee mugs full, containing as it does over 80 billion spermatozoa. In mating a zebra stallion may ejaculate as much as 300 millilitres of sperm, that is, over a quarter of a litre. After being mounted the mare appears to urinate, but in fact this is part of the seminal fluid flowing out of her body. A man discharges between 2 and 4 millilitres at each ejaculation. To put things in perspective, the volumes of a number of other animal species are as follows: bats 0.05, foxes 1.5, dogs 6, domesticated donkeys 50, domesticated horses 70, domesticated billy-goats 1 and turkeys 0.3 millilitres.

The male actually owes the scrotum to his female origin. It is only at the moment when it is decided that the embryo is to continue its development as a male that the embryonic labia grow together to form the scrotum. One has only to look closely: right down the centre of the scrotum runs a line of raised skin, the scrotal seam.

According to some experts, there is a good reason for the positioning of the testicles outside the abdominal cavity (though dissenting voices will also be heard in this book). The first group see the normal body temperature of between 36.5°C and 37°C as too high for the

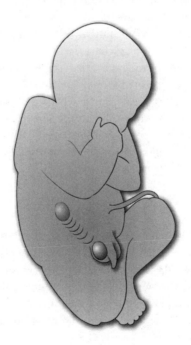

Testicular descent
in a male foetus.

efficient production, maturation and storage of healthy human sperm cells. That is the principal reason why nature has opted for a location in the cool-box that we call the scrotum, where the prevailing temperature is between 33 and 34 degrees. One way in which this cool-box operates is through vascular temperature regulation: the artery supplying warm blood from the abdominal cavity is quite convoluted just above the testicles and is surrounded by a complex network of vessels called the *plexus pampiniformis*. This network transports cool arterial blood from the testes back towards the heart. That colder blood washes around the main artery and ensures that the arterial blood flowing to the testicles is cooled so that it cannot harm the young sperm cells. The fact that testicles need protection from both excessively high and excessively low temperatures is evident from a feature that in our modern society benefits only inveterate naturists: the strong pigmentation of the skin of the scrotum. This dates from when primitive man wandered around the African savannahs without protective clothing. A dark skin after all offers more protection against sunlight than a light one. But too low a temperature is not good either! Every man who walks into the sea from a warm beach knows this: the cremaster muscles instantly lift the testes back towards the warmer groin.

The location of the testicles outside the body was therefore probably designed to protect the reproductive cells from extremes of temperature. However, one further safety measure was put in place, namely the so-called blood-testicle barrier. Sperm cells are very unusual, in more than one respect. They are haploid, that is, they contain only one copy of our genetic material. All other cells are diploid, containing a copy in duplicate of hereditary characteristics. Such diploid cells are regarded as malignant intruders in the testicles. By its own logic the immune system has an irresistible tendency to attack anything with the characteristics of a sperm cell. This is why the blood-testicle barrier, with the aid of a membrane and special Sertoli cells, seals off the sperm-producing tubes from diploid body cells. If this line of defence is breached the man will start producing antibodies against his own spermatozoa.

Animals

The testicles of the blue whale are over 70 cm long and weigh about 50 kg. Testicle dimensions in whales vary greatly, as they do in man. Yet the sperm cells of this whale are no larger than human sperm cells. Human testicles have a combined weight of approximately 40 g, corresponding to roughly 0.06 per cent of total body weight. The testicles of a stallion weigh almost 350 g, or 0.27 per cent of its total body weight.

Chimpanzees have the heaviest testicles of all anthropoid apes, with a combined weight of 119 g (0.27% of body weight), while a gorilla's testicles are much smaller, in both relative and absolute terms (29.6 g, 0.02%). The human male is therefore somewhere in the middle.

Species	Weight of testicles in grams	Percentage of body weight
man	40	0.06
chimpanzee	118.8	0.27
gorilla	29.6	0.02
orang-utan	35.3	0.05
rhesus monkey	46.2	0.50
mantle baboon	27.1	0.13
rabbit	5.5	0.13
golden hamster	0.3	0.30
water vole	3.8	0.68
wild boar	720	0.41
ram (sheep)	500	0.63
stallion (horse)	340	0.71

There is very special sub-group among fighting cocks: they have especially large testicles, and are both 'transvestites' and 'homosexual'. This type of male was discovered some years ago by a Frisian potato farmer and bird expert, Joop Jukema. The unusual creature turned out to be hard to distinguish from a female with the naked eye and displayed homosexual behaviour. The discovery was a bombshell for the biological community. The farmer christened his discovery *faar*, which in Frisian means patriarch. Only 1 per cent of the breed are patriarchs. It had been discovered fifty years previously that there are different types of fighting cock males: 'basemen', which defend a small territory against others like themselves, and 'satellites'. The latter forage about and are tolerated by the basemen. At the time this discovery caused a sensation, but finding a third type half a century later was extraordinary.

According to the potato farmer the faar was discovered so late because its appearance meant that it was mistaken for a female. Females are brown, while males have strikingly coloured neck feathers to impress females, and in addition the male is considerably larger than the female. The discoverer began to doubt the received wisdom when he occasionally spotted a bird that departed from the norm: a fighting cock without spectacular neck feathers, but with the dimensions of a male. As regards colour it was a female, but the wings were over 17 cm long, which was very unusual for a female. Internal examination showed it to be a male, with particularly large testicles. Of course the farmer called in back-up, from scientists at Groningen University. There was great curiosity about the faar's reproductive behaviour: it was found to have a preference for mating with its own sex.

The researchers assumed that the faars 'leave their sperm behind' in basemen, which then transfer it to a female. Thanks to their large testicles they can easily swamp sperm from other males with their abundant production. Normally they have little chance of mating with a female, because females are closely guarded by other males. These homosexual 'transvestites' are not inclined to compete openly, and yet have found a way of reproducing!

A comparable situation exists with lizards of the genus *anolis*. Some males remain as small as females and hence are not regarded as rivals by other males. They are able to move about the territory of larger male lizards unnoticed and mate with females. They must, though, keep a low profile, or they run the risk of unwanted homosexual contact.

Numbers tell the tale

The volume of a testicle can be estimated by using a tape measure and comparing the readings with plastic models of known volume. For adult men the volume usually exceeds 15 millilitres. A volume of between 17 and 25 millilitres is regarded as normal. The length varies from 3 to 6 cm, the width from 2 to over 3 cm. Large or small, these glands constitute an extremely ingenious production unit which every day turns out between ten and a hundred million 'homunculi', or tiny male creatures.

The volume and firmness of the testicle may indicate whether there are any endocrinal abnormalities. Small, rubbery testicles in a grown man, for example, may indicate insufficient stimulation. Before puberty the testicles are small, but the absence of a testicle from the scrotum is abnormal. It may be a case of a retractile testicle caused by the tensing of the testicular muscles, whereby the testicle is pulled in the direction of the external inguinal opening or even the inguinal canal. The medical term for this phenomenon is the cremaster reflex, which causes the sudden disappearance of the testicle!

The cremaster reflex may be triggered, for example, by stimulating the skin on the inside of the upper thigh. In older men the reaction is harder to provoke. The spiral-shaped fibres of the cremaster muscles run through the seminal cord to the base of the penis and when suddenly contracted may even result in testicular torsion. On the underside the testicle is attached to the scrotum by a wide band which normally prevents it from it turning vertically on its own axis.

During sexual arousal engorgement with blood causes the testicle to increase in volume by up to 50 per cent. In the case of prolonged sexual arousal the accumulation of blood may cause pain ('blue balls'), from which ejaculation brings relief. (Not that women should feel in any way responsible for this state of affairs!) Scientists in the German state of Thüringen were able to demonstrate that when the testicles of male ferrets swelled in spring, their brains also increased in size – definitely not the case in humans!

Moving balls also seem to be an object of particular fascination for visual artists. Joop van Lieshout, for example, has produced a series of huge plastic penises, and in a TV programme he showed an excerpt from a work by his fellow-artist Bruce Nauman, who in 1969 filmed the dangling and bouncing of his own testicles with a high-speed camera, as part of a series of four *Slo Mo* films: *Black Balls*, *Bouncing Balls*, *Pulling Mouth* and *Gauze*.

Nauman hired an industrial camera to film at very high speeds: the frame speed varied from 1,000 to 4,000 per second (the normal speed is 24 FPS), in natural light. The shooting time was between four and six seconds, but the running time of *Bouncing Balls* is nine minutes. The extreme slow-motion effect means that movement is sometimes scarcely perceptible.

Leydig and Sertoli cells

Each of the two testicles – separated from each other in the scrotum by a membrane, the septum – is made up of two compartments. In terms of volume 95 per cent of the testicle is devoted to sperm production. There are approximately 250 lobules, and if you were to lay all the tubes in the lobules end to end they would have a combined length of about 500 metres. The inner wall of the tubes contains germ cells which after a process of divisions produce young but not yet mature sperm cells. Between ten and a hundred million sperm cells are produced every day.

The unbelievably dense network of fine seminal tubes constituting the sperm-producing section of the testicles was described in the seventeenth century by Reinier de Graaf, though the actual discovery was made by De Graaf's teacher, Professor Johannes van Horne of Leiden University. During a study placement in France De Graaf had used bull's testicles for his research. These were easily obtainable, but turned out to be less than ideal for research purposes. He finally opted for the testicles of an unusual little creature, the dormouse. Its body weight is approximately 100 g and the testicles weigh about 1 g each. De Graaf removed the outer membrane from the dormice testicles and then submerged them in a glass of water. When the glass was gently shaken the testicles simply fell to pieces. 'One can clearly see that the testicles consist wholly of tiny tubes,' wrote De Graaf in his book (Van Horne had previously stated that the testicle was nothing but 'a collection of tiny threads'). This was in fact plagiarism by De Graaf, but after a long correspondence with the Royal Society he was credited with the discovery of the 'threads'. For the sake of completeness he even had to forward a dissected dormouse testicle that he had preserved in alcohol.

Back to anatomy. Between the tubes, the 'threads' in which the sperm cells are formed, there are blood vessels, the Sertoli cells and the Leydig cells. The Sertoli cells, the support cells, form part of the blood-testicle barrier, controlling the emergence of the mature sperm cells: all nutriment for the maturing spermatozoa must first pass through them.

The Italian physiologist Enrico Sertoli (1842–1910) was still a medical student when he observed these 'nurse' cells in 1862. In the young embryo they make the Anti-Müllerian hormone (the Müllerian duct produces female sex organs, the Wolffian duct male ones), which ensures that the male embryo actually acquires normal sexual characteristics. After puberty the Sertoli cells produce the hormone inhibine.

The Leydig cells, named after the German anatomist Franz von Leydig (1842–1910), make up approximately 5 per cent of the total volume of the testicles, and use cholesterol to produce, from puberty onwards, about 7 milligrams per day of the male sex hormone testosterone. They do this in response to the LH (luteinizing hormone) transmitted by the hypophysis or pituitary gland at the base of the brain.

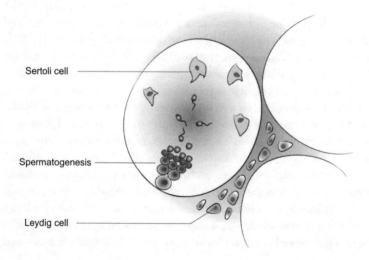

Sertoli cell

Spermatogenesis

Leydig cell

Microscopic image of testicular tissue.

The course of the
ductus ferens.

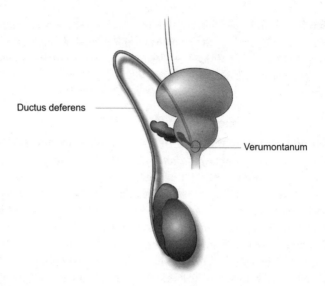

Ductus deferens

Verumontanum

Another regulating substance transmitted by the hypophysis is the Follicle Stimulating Hormone (FSH), which regulates sperm cell formation.

The seminal duct (the *ductus deferens,* or *vas deferens*) runs for a distance of between 30 and 40 cm from the epididymis to the *verumontanum*, an elevation or crest in the wall of the urethra in the centre of the prostate.

Also near the prostate, behind the bladder, are the two seminal glands (*vesiculae seminalis*), which despite what their name suggests do not store sperm cells but produce fluid, part of the transport medium for the sperm cells. After all, in an ejaculation it is not only sperm cells that are expelled. An ejaculate consists in large part of fluid originating from the seminal glands and the prostate. The sperm cells account for only a small percentage of the total volume. In older medical literature a distinction is made between the section of the sperm cell constituting the 'noblest part', the 'aqueous elements' from the seminal glands, and the 'oleagenous' section from the prostate.

In the late 1950s Japanese researchers conducted experiments with x-ray contrast media that showed clearly how the different sections emerged. First sperm cells were forced from the epididymis in the direction of the ampoule of the seminal duct. The ampoule is a protuberance close to the spot where the seminal duct discharges, in which a quantity of sperm can be stored. Then the muscles around the seminal glands contract, and the sperm cells with fluid originating from the seminal glands are forced together into the prostatic section of the urethra, where they are mixed with prostate liquid. One striking feature is that some sperm cells also return to the ampoule and seminal glands.

The seminal glands particularly contain many nooks and crannies where sperm cells can linger for a considerable period. A practical result of this is that for a long time after sterilization sperms may sometimes be visible in the ejaculate.

The smell and taste of sperm

Women often compare the smell of sperm to plant or flower scents. Herb Robert (*Geranium robertianum*), St John's wort (*Hypericum perforatum*), the flowers of the European barberry (*Berberis vulgaris*) and chestnuts all smell of sperm. The same applies to the crushed flowers of the henna plant (*Lawsonia inermis*). Moroccan women love rubbing them into their palms, while Western European women use them, often in powder form, to dye their hair.

Billy-goats, long regarded as the epitome of animal horniness, spray their own beards with sperm and urine. The Ancient Greeks dreamt up all kinds of hybrids of man and billy-goat, such as the demi-god Satyr and the forest god Pan, and the physical attributes of these sensuous figures (horns, hoofs and beard) were adopted by Christianity to depict the Devil. Billy-goats, however, have some surprisingly female aspects. If one massages their nipples for an extended period, a milk-giving udder appears in front of the scrotum!

The American jazz musician Charles Mingus compared the texture of sperm to cream: 'She gulps and slurps the cream out of me while I melt and she sucks hard at my tree.' John Hunter, a nineteenth-century English surgeon, observed in one of his essays that 'if one holds sperm in one's mouth it gives a warmth like spices'. The celebrated sexologist Havelock Ellis (1859–1939) wrote that many primitive peoples, particularly the Australian aborigines, made potions from sperm, which were given to sick or dying members of the tribe. In addition he mentions the Manicheans and the Albigensians, who sprinkled the bread used for Holy Communion with human sperm. In the seventeenth century sperm was regarded as an effective defence against witchcraft and a precious aphrodisiac. The church, however, refused to tolerate it, and in his book Ellis records prison sentences of seven years for the offence.

According to reliable sources it is not unusual for young women today in a get-together in the pub to admit whether they 'swallow' or not. They're not talking about E, amphetamines or suchlike, but whether or not they swallow sperm. There is some similarity between suckling and fellatio, between mother's milk and sperm: just as an infant can taste whether its mother has eaten garlic, a woman who 'swallows' can taste the garlic that her partner has eaten the day before. Sperm is both stronger in flavour and more bitter if a man smokes and drinks a lot of coffee, while the sperm of vegetarians reputedly tastes better than that of carnivores. Kiwi fruit particularly are supposed to improve the flavour. A famous (male) Dutch comic duo felt that truly emancipated women should immediately spit the sperm out again. I can't remember why, nor do I have any ready-made answer on the subject. I do know, though, that only three men in every thousand can suck themselves off.

While we are talking about ejaculation and secretion, this is the place to mention in passing the glands about which the English physician William Cowper was the first to publish in 1702, situated a little upstream of the prostate and also issuing into the urethra, which in a state of arousal produce the so-called preseminal fluid. In women the corresponding glands are named after the Danish researcher Bartholin (1585–1629).

The smell of the scrotum

The degree of hirsuteness and the smell of the scrotum vary – a topic that was raised as early as the 1870s in the work of the American feminist novelist and campaigner Lois Waisbrooker (1826–1909). Some of today's racy pulp novelists, one feels, should have been made to study Erica Jong's *Fear of Flying* (1974) as prescribed reading. In the latter book, with disarming frankness and great literary panache, Jong (1942–) evokes the physical attributes of her lovers, ephemeral and more significant:

> I once adored a conductor who never bathed, had stringy hair, and was a complete failure at wiping his ass. He always left shit stripes on my sheets. Normally I don't go in for that sort of thing – but in him it was OK – I'm still not sure why. I fell in love with Bennett partly because he had the cleanest balls I'd ever tasted. Hairless and he practically never sweats. You could (if you wanted) eat off his asshole (like my grandmother's kitchen floor).

And later:

> We lay on his bed and held each other. We examined each other's nakedness with tenderness and amusement. The best thing about making love with a new man after all those years of marriage was rediscovering a man's body. One's husband's body was practically like one's own. Everything about it was known. All the smells and tastes of it, the lines, the hairs, the

birthmarks. But Adrian was like a new country. My tongue made an unguided tour of it. I started at his mouth and went downward. His broad neck, which was sun-burned. His chest, covered with curly reddish hair. His belly, a bit paunchy – unlike Bennett's brown leanness. His curled pink penis which tasted vaguely of urine and refused to stand up in my mouth. His very pink and hairy balls which I took in my mouth one at a time.

The technique Erica Jong is referring to here is called 'teabagging'. The partner takes the testicles in his or her mouth – the testicles are first pushed downwards with the index finger and thumb around the top of the scrotum, and then the balls are taken into the mouth and gently stimulated with the tongue. The teeth are covered with the lips throughout, to avoid accidentally inflicting pain. The testicles are kept together; if they are pulled apart, it can be dreadfully painful.

Dartos

Back to temperature regulation by the scrotum: the skin of the scrotum is characterized, like that of the eyelids, by the absence of subcutaneous fat, the presence of many tiny blood vessels, and a layer of muscle directly under the skin. Fat insulates too well, which does not help the ability to react rapidly to cold or heat. The muscular layer beneath the skin is called the *tunica dartos*. As we grow older the *tunica dartos* slackens, so that in elderly men the scrotum becomes larger and smoother. Everything starts to hang: it comes to resemble a set of bells. In cold temperatures the scrotum shrinks and when it is hot the muscle layer relaxes and the scrotum expands.

'Croat traps testicles in sun lounger', read a recent newspaper headline. Trying to stand up and finding to your annoyance that your testicles are trapped between the slats of your lounger is no joke. But it happened to Mario Visnjic after he had swum naked around the harbour of Valalta (Western Croatia). Mario had no inkling of danger when he sat down in his chair to get his breath back after his cold dip. The cold sea had caused his testicles to shrink, so that they dropped between the wooden slats of the lounger. When a little later the sun did its work and the testicles expanded to their true size again, the damage was done. His rescuer had no alternative but to cut the lounger in half and release the unfortunate victim!

The blood supply to the scrotum is through the large inguinal artery, the deep pelvic artery and the abdominal wall artery. Lymphatic drainage takes place through the superficial lymph glands in the groin.

It is important for the reader with hypochondriac tendencies to know exactly how lymphatic drainage works: this will help doctors to know exactly where to look for metastases.

The skin of the scrotum is fairly sensitive. Delicate nerve-endings are designed to maximize pleasure. Swellings on the skin of the scrotum are almost always sebaceous cysts. Treatment is necessary only if there is an infection. Swellings of the content of the scrotum, the testicles and epididymis are much more common. Various sections will be devoted to these in later chapters.

The blood supply to the testicles is closely related to that to the kidneys because of their common embryological origin. The main artery in the testicle (*arteria testicularis*) branches off the aorta just below the renal artery. The artery runs behind the abdominal cavity through the inguinal canal to the testicle. There are connections to the seminal duct artery. The latter is a branch of the main inguinal artery. In the seminal cord there is a tangle of arteries (*plexus pampiniformis*), from where blood flows back to the heart. On a level with the internal ring of the inguinal canal this complex becomes the drainage vein (*vena spermatica interna*). On the right-hand side this flows directly into the inferior vena cava, and on the left into the renal vein. This division is the reason why varicose veins in the scrotum, varicocele, are much more common on the left than on the right.

Lymphatic drainage from the testicles is in the first instance into lymph glands behind the abdomen and not, as many people think, into glands in the groin. That fact is particularly important in the treatment of testicular cancer. The lymph glands in the groin do, however, form part of the drainage system of lymph from the skin of the scrotum. In the past cancer of the skin of the scrotum was very common among chimney sweeps and coalmen, who had soot and coal dust more or less continually in their crotch. Today cancer of the skin of the scrotum is extremely rare.

Nerve supply

A dentist about to start root canal work on a woman suddenly feels her hand firmly grasping his testicles. As he stares at the women open-mouthed, she says with a smile: 'Let's promise not to hurt each other!' Pain in the testicles is excruciating, but hard to understand even for doctors. The fact is that nerve provision in the testes is complicated. The autonomous, sympathetic nerve supply derives from the spinal segments of the tenth and twelfth vertebrae. These nerves run parallel with the blood vessels. They penetrate the fibrous sheath surrounding the testicles (*tunica albuginea*) and continue their course among the lobules

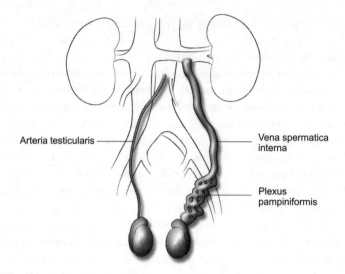

Arteria testicularis

Vena spermatica interna

Plexus pampiniformis

The plexus pampiniformis and the vena spermatica inferma.

where the sperm cells are produced. Their most important function seems to be to affect the contraction or otherwise of the smooth muscular tissue in the tunica albuginea. The nerve endings governing sensation in the testicles are located in the same compartment as the Leydig cells. If the skin of the scrotum and the *tunica vaginalis* are anaesthetized and the testicle is then injected with a physiological salt solution, pain is felt not in the scrotum, but instead deep down in the abdomen. This is probably referred pain, deriving from the autonomous nerve supply.

The somatic, or non-autonomous nerve supply is through the *nervus genito-femoralis* and derives from the spinal segments of the first and second lumbar vertebrae. The nerve branch to the interior of the scrotum runs first to the testicular muscles, and passes right through them before continuing to the tunica vaginalis and tunica albuginea of the testicles. If in the course of an operation this nerve is severed, whether or not deliberately, henceforth when the testicles are squeezed hard pain will be felt only deep in the groin. With spinal anaesthesia up to the level of the first lumbar vertebrae 'testicle sensation' also disappears. The above findings indicate that only with intense stimulation, for example hard squeezing, does autonomous nerve pain occur: dull, nauseating pain that is difficult to localize. If pain is clearly felt in the scrotum, it is conducted via somatic nerves.

Referred pain in the scrotum may be the result of, for example, a kidney stone that has descended into the urethra, a weak spot in the inguinal artery, a minute hernia in the groin that is not yet visible or wear and tear on the spinal column.

The epididymis

The sperm-forming tubes in a testicle discharge into a kind of transit depot. Between six and eight ducts lead to the epididymis. In the epididymis those ducts merge into a single tube. While the sperm-forming tubes in a testicle have a combined length of 250 metres, an epididymis is a duct of approximately 6 metres in length. The epididymis curls in a comma-shape behind the testicle. One can distinguish a head (*caput*), a body (*corpus*) and a tail (*cauda*). On a level with the head of the epididymis the network of drainage tubes in the testicle connects to the narrow epididymal duct, and the tail then connects to the seminal duct, the *ductus deferens*.

The blood supply comes both from the testicular artery and from its own epididymal artery. Drainage of blood takes place through the previously mentioned *plexus pampiniformis*. During a passage of several days through the epididymis the still infertile sperm cells mature into fertile cells. One of the most striking changes is an increase in the percentage of moving spermatozoa and their swimming speed. Biochemical changes in their surface increase the ability of sperm cells to attach themselves to the ovum.

The epididymis is highly dependent on testosterone, and the head is exposed to high concentrations through the influx from the testicles. Further down stream in the epididymis, the concentration of testosterone is much lower. Besides the testosterone supply via the *rete testis* (testicular network of tubes), the epididymis is also supplied with testosterone via the bloodstream. The exposure of different sections of

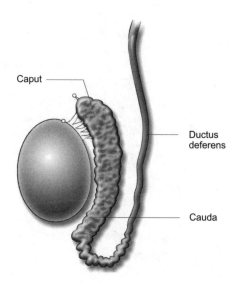

Caput

Ductus deferens

Cauda

The epididymis.

the epididymis to different concentrations of testosterone make it a unique organ.

At orgasm the sperm cell stored in the tail of the epididymis are forced into the seminal duct. The impetus is provided by the contraction of the smooth muscles in the wall of this long, tubular organ. If a man does not ejaculate for two weeks, sperm cells will appear spontaneously in his urine.

The seminal duct

The ductus deferens, between 30 and 40 cm long, links the epididymis with the urethra. Immediately before the actual ejaculation rhythmic contractions take place in the smooth muscle tissue of the wall, propelling the sperm cells towards the ampoule and the urethra. This muscle-lined tube with a diameter of between 3 and 4 mm can be felt between the tail of the epididymis and the external groin opening. It feels like a liquorice shoelace. In this area the duct forms part of the seminal cord, which also consists of arteries and a network of veins, nerves and lymph vessels.

The seminal cord is encased in structures originating from the abdominal wall, the *fascia spermatica interna* and the *fascia spematica externa*. Contained in this casing are the cremaster or transverse testicular muscles. From the inner inguinal ring the seminal duct runs along the inside of the abdominal wall, passing behind the bladder to the centre of the prostate. Close to the prostate, between the bladder

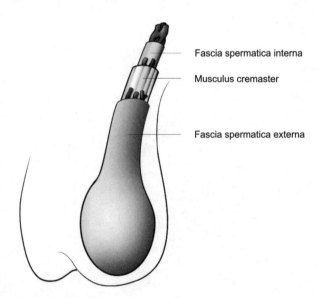

Fascia spermatica interna

Musculus cremaster

Fascia spermatica externa

The covering of the seminal cord.

The appendices
of the testicle and
the epididymis.

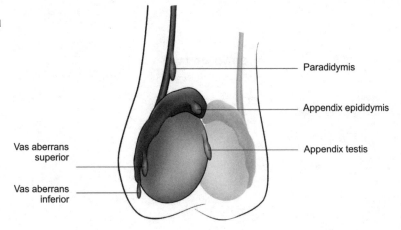

Paradidymis

Appendix epididymis

Appendix testis

Vas aberrans
superior

Vas aberrans
inferior

and the rectum, the duct widens into the ampoule (*ampulla ductus deferentis*). Within the prostate the duct narrows to the ejaculatory duct, or *ductus ejaculatorius*. The two ejaculatory ducts discharge at a point near the *verumontanum*, a thickening in the rear wall of the urethra that runs right through the prostate.

Appendices

Attached to the testicle and the epididymis are a number of appendices that are polyp-shaped, up to 1 cm long and up to 2 cm in diameter. These are: the *appendix testis* (Morgagni's hydatid), the *appendix epididymis*, the *paradidymis* (organ of Giraldis), the *superior vas aberrans superior* (Haller's organ) and the *vas aberrans inferior*.

An appendix testis is found in 90 per cent of men. It originates from remnants of Müller's duct, a structure in the embryo from which female sex organs are made. The other appendices (remnants of mesonephric tubules) are much less common. An appendix to the epididymis is found in 30 per cent of men, the last three mentioned in a maximum of between 1 and 5 per cent. Torsion can result in acute pain in these organs – nearly always in the appendix testis – and in the atrophy of the appendix. There is, though, absolutely no need for an operation in such cases.

chapter two

The Penis

Impotence means literally the inability to perform sexual intercourse, though the word is often used in a disparaging sense, implying helplessness. Impotence is probably one of the best kept bedroom secrets and, at least for those affected, one of the most shameful. Fortunately a euphemism has been devised: erection problems or, even more useful, erectile dysfunction or ED.

Modern medicine sees the erection of the penis as based on a neurovascular reflex, dependent on a correct hormonal balance, a healthy anatomy, an adequate blood supply and an undamaged and efficiently functioning nervous system. If one takes all this on board, one realizes that it's easy for things to go wrong occasionally. Put more strongly, it's a miracle that things go smoothly so often! So this chapter will highlight not only the technical, but also the miraculous aspects.

Displaying an erection or having sex in public is not usually possible – in fact, it's illegal. So to show that one is functioning properly as a man, there is only one option, which is to father a child. If that fails, for example because of poor sperm quality, the man involved feels seriously inadequate. These days things are a little less pressured, since quite a few married couples opt – by their own testimony, at least – for voluntary childlessness. (This topic will be discussed in greater depth later.)

There has never been such a thing as an impotent woman. Leaving aside anatomical or mental abnormalities, every woman is capable of passively accepting a man's sexual advances. This is sadly not true of the man, and for that reason a man's relationship with his penis is not comparable with a woman's with her clitoris and/or vagina. A woman says 'I'm not in the mood'; for her the vagina is an integral part of her body. Of course a man's penis is too, but an erect penis, the phallus, is more.

In the novel *Io e lui* (1971, English title *The Two of Us*) by the Italian writer Alberto Moravia, the hero Federico is constantly getting into difficult and embarrassing situations because of his huge and demanding penis, which he calls Federico Rex. It is a confrontational book: the protagonist is constantly debating with his unruly member and plunging into every conceivable erotic folly. The final scene is humiliating for Federico: his member, 'he', carries him back triumphantly to the woman from whom he had tried to escape:

> To satisfy him, I pressed the bell once more. Standing stiffly in the air, 'he' seemed now to be rising up, in short, successive jerks, as if to bring himself to the level of the keyhole and look into the flat. At last I heard a slight bustling sound. Then Fausta's voice asking: 'Who is it?'
> 'It's me, Rico.'
> Fausta's hand undid the chain, the door opened, and she appeared on the threshold in her dressing-gown. She looked at me, looked down, saw 'him' and then, without saying a word, put out her hand to take hold of 'him', as one might take hold of a donkey's halter to make it move. Then she turned her back to me, pulling 'him' in behind her, and, with 'him', me. She went into the flat; 'he' went behind her: I followed them both.

The title of the novel is very apt, in both Italian and English. Many men suspect or think that their penis has a will of its own and does what it likes. Quite a few men refer to their penis as 'he'. It is the symbol of the ability to procreate with the accompanying feelings of male self-worth. Muscularity, determination, effectiveness, penetration, directness, strength – the phallus underlies them all.

And so it happens that every man discovers one fine day that his penis is not like an arm, finger or leg: it doesn't react automatically. The penis can be compared to a well-trained dog, which usually follows the instructions it is given – but the owner must always allow for the possibility that one day it will refuse, despite the fact that it is trained, or in more human terms, socialized. Men can gain some control over their penis: on a nudist beach, for example, you scarcely ever see men with erections, although there are naked women (or men) to admire everywhere. A half-naked woman lying in stirrups for a bladder examination is unlikely to provoke an erection in any urologist. He is focused on the sick woman in front of him.

The phallus

Phallus is the name given to the erect penis as a symbol; most people associate the term penis with something or someone else, for example their bearded biology teacher from school or sex education manuals. This is not to say that the sex education manuals of, say, the 1960s were bad books – on the contrary, they preserved some of the mystery surrounding the adolescent penis. Their modern counterparts are so intrusive that little is left to the imagination. One of the nicest things about puberty is surely discovering things for yourself and making your own mind up. Fortunately for most young children the discovery of the differences between the male and female external sex organs is still a very exciting business. Who has never played 'doctors and nurses'? In such situations the differences are discussed at length, something that most adults no longer do or dare to do. In his fascinating novel *The Year of Cancer* (1972) the Flemish writer Hugo Claus shows that it can sometimes still happen.

> 'You've got the nicest pussy I've ever seen,' he whispered.
>
> 'No,' she said. 'It used to be nice. But when I had the baby they stitched me up wrong. And afterwards I got piles. It often hurts really badly.'
>
> 'I love you,' said Pierre.
>
> 'I love you,' she said. 'And you've got the nicest one I've ever seen too. I don't usually look at them with men.'
>
> 'But if you've never looked, how do you know mine's nicer?'
>
> 'Well, I have sneaked a look. Most of them are red or bluish. Ugh!'

The girl in this story emphasizes a common female view of the penis. With the phallus it is a different story, for men too. In many ancient cultures the phallus was the symbol of immortality, of vitality eternally renewing itself. It was no accident that at the end of his life the celebrated English writer D. H. Lawrence was fascinated by the Etruscans, who placed a phallus on every grave. As an outwardly visible biological feature the phallus came in the course of history to bear a heavy religious and moral burden. Consequently the study of the phallus led to the study of theology, of the phallus that rises and when the party is over dies again, and that as an 'immortal' can repeat this feat again and again: the eternal resurrection of the flesh.

The phallus cult was a striking feature of Ancient Greek religion, and the impotent man was more mocked than pitied. For the Greeks a small phallus was preferable, since a large one was associated with barbarians and satyrs. That may have been connected with Aristotle's view that a shorter penis enhanced fertility. He thought that 'sperm cools down less the shorter the distance to be travelled'.

Both in front of temples and at the doors of Athenian homes there stood a herm, a square column with a man's head and an erect penis at the front, but without limbs. Herms stood not only in front of homes, but also at city gates, outside citadels, in markets and in gymnasiums. In short, they were everywhere in Ancient Greece. The herm was wreathed in green and had olive oil poured over it. During worship people put their hand on its head, or took hold of it by the beard or the phallus. The latter action particularly would not be possible nowadays. But wait a minute! In Piazza Signoria in Florence there is a Neptune in the middle of a pool, around which are a number of seated bronze fauns all naked and with erect penises. Although for the most part the bronze of the fauns has the familiar oxidized colour, the phalluses are like brass, due to the countless hands that have taken them by that part of the body and stroked them. Florentine women believe that this increases their chances of becoming pregnant. But what a difference: while the touching in Florence takes place in secret, in Ancient Greek it happened freely and publicly. Sexuality and religious observance were inseparable. Of course, the symbolic significance of the phallus embraced much more than sex alone. At Dionysian celebrations its religious importance was stressed, and huge phalluses were borne in procession. Dionysus was the god of intoxication, of the ecstatic rapture brought about by wine, the blood of the earth, the god of passion and of the rowdy exuberance that characterized these autumnal festivities.

In the drama *Acharnes* the Greek comic playwright Aristophanes (*c.*446–*c.*386 BC) tells the story of the procession marking the private Dionysian celebration held by the good Dikaiopolis together with his daughter and his slave Xanthius on the occasion of the armistice between Athens and Sparta. In advance of the procession he instructs Xanthius to hold the phallus pole straight in front of him, and then sings the following phallic hymn:

> Oh, Phales, companion of Bacchus,
> life of the party, old goat,
> lover of women and boys,
> with peace in my hands I greet you
> and rejoicing return to my village.

The great city festivals of Dionysus were important civic events. They were accompanied by much pomp and ceremony and drew spectators from miles around. Not only were countless phallic images carried in procession, but the participants also tied on large artificial penises.

However, it was precisely the Greeks who drew a sharp line between the phallus in its symbolic meaning and the same organ as an anatomical component. The phallus was used only symbolically and ritually.

An Egyptian creation story tells of the primordial god Atum, who created the world by masturbating while standing in the primeval sea, encouraged by Hathor, the goddess of love: from his phallus he spewed Shu and Tefnet, the god of air and the goddess of liquid, brother and sister, and with that creation was complete. Moreover, in Egyptian mythology there was a god of male sexual power. His name was Min and he was of some importance. He is usually depicted with his left hand round his phallus and his right hand raised in an inverted v-shaped structure, supposedly representing coitus.

In the Hindu creation myth a phallus is also described. In 1959 Paul Thomas devoted a book to the subject: on the day of their creation, when the gods Brahma and Vishi appeared out of nowhere, they were bewildered, but 'soon they saw a dazzling lingam of huge proportions, whose extremities reached vast distances'.

The phallus also played an important role in the religion of other ancient peoples. Not only in Baal worship (Baal was the phallic god of the Canaanites), but in Islam and Judaism too the circumcision of the foreskin became a sign of the link between the man and Baal, Allah and Jahweh respectively.

It is worth mentioning that in chapter 20 of the Old Testament book of Deuteronomy, which concerns those who shall not enter into the congregation of the Lord, there is mention of 'he that is wounded in the stones [testicles], or hath his privy member cut off'. Obviously such injuries were a problem even then.

According to the etymologist G. R. Scott the Bible translators deliberately replaced the word 'penis' with the euphemism 'hip' and later 'loin' or 'thigh'. An obvious example is found in Genesis 24:2–3, where Abraham addresses his eldest servant: 'Put, I pray thee, thy hand under my thigh: and I will make thee swear by the Lord, the God of heaven, and the God of the earth, that thou shalt not take a wife unto my son . . .' In Abraham's time it was simply the custom when swearing an oath to touch one's own penis or the penis of the person most closely involved. The circumcised member, after all, was the sign of the bond between man and Jehovah.

In Christianity the penis gradually faded into the background as a religious symbol, although traditionally, especially in France, powers for the cure of impotence were attributed to certain saints down to the end of the nineteenth century. In one's hour of need one could address one's prayers to them.

Until 1805, when the village was buried by an earthquake, a picturesque pilgrimage took place annually on 17 September in Isernia (near Naples). In the cathedral the relics of St Damien were displayed. On the great day these were carried in procession to the local fair. Wax phalluses of every shape and size were on sale, and worshippers were required to hang one in the chapel while intoning a particular prayer. The proceeds of course went to the church. There were many other places where the Catholic Church sanctioned phallus worship, more details may be found in *A History of Phallic Worship* by R. Payne Knight and T. Wright.

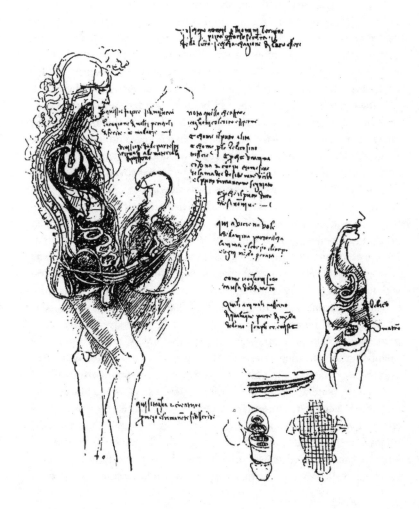

Leonardo da Vinci's cross-section of a fornicating couple.

The beginnings of science

One of the first people to study the penis and erection scientifically was Leonardo da Vinci. The most incisive mind in human history took a keen interest in the sexual organs.

In his view the genitalia both of the man and of the woman were so repulsive that, were it not for the beauty of the human body as a whole and irrepressible sexual desire, the human race would long since have died out. Through his anatomical studies Leonardo fell foul of the ban on dissecting corpses. This brilliant man – with a personal erotic preference for his own sex – refuted the medieval notion that an erection came about as a result of an accumulation of air. After research on hanged criminals, he rightly concluded that erections in man were caused by an accumulation of blood.

However, this is not the case with all mammals. In birds, for example, erection results from lymph congestion. Not surprisingly, the vast majority of such creatures are not in possession of a real penis, that is, an organ containing masses of erectile tissue. Only the Ratitae, including ostriches, and the Anseres (swans, geese and ducks, which copulate under water) have penises containing erectile tissue. The Argentine duck has a penis that when fully erect averages 43 cm in length, making it longer than the duck itself. What's more, this bird not only has a huge penis, but also turns out to have a very active and promiscuous sex life – too beastly for words. The assumption that the duck's enormous penis was aimed at attracting females proved incorrect. It is simply a well-hung species that not even the ostrich can match.

If any reader is ever in Iceland, I would advise them to drop in at the Phallological Museum in Reykjavík, the only one of its kind. Every normal utilitarian object is here remodelled in the shape of a penis. The handle of a door, the strong box, the pens, everything. In addition there is an exhibition of 137 penises from forty different species. The largest is that of a sperm whale, and measures 1.7 metres. The museum is also hoping for a penis from Homo sapiens. Whatever happens it seems sure of acquiring one, since three men have promised to leave their manhood to the museum after their death. A wax impression of the member of one of them is already hanging on display. Meanwhile the geysers continue to arouse great interest with their spouts of steam . . .

The anatomist Costanzo Varolio (1543–1575) wrote about erection some decades after Leonardo. One of his conclusions was that the erection was the result of a *stase* of blood. In his view muscles on the underside of the penis played a major role. The scholar Reinier de Graaf from Delft, discussed above, had invented a type of syringe with which he carried out many different kinds of research on dead

The long
corkscrew penis
of the Argentine
duck.

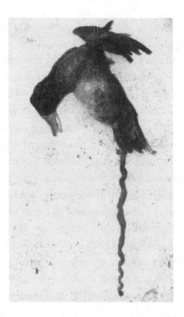

bodies. To his amazement, when he injected the *arteria hypogastrica* he saw the erectile tissue in the penis filling up, confirming Varolio's conclusion.

In 1668 De Graaf completed his study of the male sex organ. He rushed the report to the printer together with an article on the use of enemas and anatomical injections, so anxious was he to pip his teacher, Leiden professor Johannes van Horne, to the post. De Graaf was well aware that the male sex organ was a tricky subject, since 'disrespectful, lewd people will try to misuse what I publish for wanton images and smutty jokes'. His defence was that he had presented his finding in as decent a way as possible, so that 'no one can take the slightest offence, unless they are determined to do so'. De Graaf's book, with the catchy title *De virorum inservientibus, de clysteribus et de usu siphonis in anatomi* (Treatise on the Reproductive Organs, and the Use of the Hypodermic Syringe in Anatomy), contained a summary of the anatomy of the penis, but also a description of his method of injecting cadavers with ink in order to make the blood vessels visible.

De Graaf was born in 1641 to Roman Catholic parents. His mother came from a wealthy family and his father was a successful ship-builder. Although Catholics were allowed to practise their religion in the Dutch Republic, the state was Protestant and De Graaf had no prospect of ever becoming a professor. The young prodigy, who must have realized from an early age that he belonged to a minority, first attended the Catholic University of Leuven, before moving on to a preparatory course at the University of Utrecht, and in 1663 went to

Leiden to study medicine. Matthew Cobb, in his book *The Egg and Sperm Race*, creates a vivid picture of student life at this period. In his view it was remarkably similar to that of the twenty-first century, although there were no female students. Students lived in cramped quarters, sometimes ten to a house, and just as today often changed addresses. Student life consisted of study, drink, dancing till the small hours, and sex. Every social event was an excuse for getting drunk, and the university authorities actually encouraged the consumption of alcohol, promising would-be students an annual tax-free alcohol allowance of 194 litres of wine and approximately 1,500 litres of beer! In the smoky taverns medical students were often teased about the bad reputation of their intended profession. 'We don't need a doctor, we'd rather die for nothing,' was a typical dig.

Reinier de Graaf died aged only 32. Nothing is known about the cause of his death, but over twenty years later Antonie van Leeuwenhoek claimed to have heard at the time that he had been taken ill after an altercation with his scientific rival Jan Swammerdam.

Back to the main story. In 1863 the German physiologist Conrad Eckhardt (1822–1905) demonstrated that an erection could be induced by stimulating the sacrum. The erection centre was located in the lowest part of the spine – that much was certain – but it was to be a long time before any more became known about the process. Even at the time when Neil Armstrong walked on the moon, we still had only a vague notion. In the 1940s German researchers discovered that not only adult men but also male babies have nocturnal erections. So obviously such erections are not in themselves linked to testosterone levels, which after all only start to rise in puberty. In the 1950s equipment was gradually designed for the objective measurement of erections. Naturally such advances were abused: in Czechoslovakia an erection meter served to expose men pretending to be gay in order to avoid national service. The recruits were shown hard-core hetero porn while attached to an erection meter, and quickly gave the game away!

In Britain the erection meter was still in use in the 1990s, but in the psychiatric assessment of long-term sex offenders. The prison psychiatrists showed their patients perverse or violent videos, while the sensors hidden in the tapes that had been attached to their penises gave an accurate record of whether or not they were still aroused. In the case of arousal their release into society was delayed. Only a short while ago I was approached about using a similar diagnostic method experimentally . . .

Sometimes it is the patient himself who insists on nocturnal erection readings. An example is a 42-year-old man accused of having sexual relations with his stepdaughter. The court had already sentenced him to several months' imprisonment. However, he maintained to his lawyer, his GP and myself that he had been impotent for years and for that reason could not be guilty. He wanted this confirmed and hence was briefly admitted to hospital for nocturnal erection monitoring. The readings were normal, and that was the end of that.

The shrinking penis

The fact that in the distant past there were so many different ways of delivering sperm cells – with some male animals surpassing others by developing methods of getting as close as possible to the ovum – led to the evolution of the penis. It was to play a crucial role in reproduction.

There are many different kinds of penis: the *aedeagus* of flies, mites and butterflies, the protuberances that some frogs have near their anus, the tiny organ with which the drone of the common-or-garden bee copulates (it breaks off and costs the drone its life, but does prevent others from mating with the queen), the *embolus* of the golden spider, the anal fin of fishes, the double penises of snakes, the proboscis of the dragonfly. Ostriches are particularly well equipped, and at the turn of the twentieth century walking sticks were made from their penises. Male organs vary from little protuberances to whale penises, which, though they are usually hidden in the body, can reach a length of almost 2 metres. In the fearsome cold encountered on an expedition to find the North-East Passage led by Willem Barentsz in 1596, the ship's doctor tanned the only part of a whale's skin that is fit for tanning and made it into a waistcoat. Calvinist that he was, he had his Bible bound in the same material – penis leather. The phallus, death and religion are, after all, closely connected.

Leather can also be obtained from the human penis. Sceptics should visit Wieuwerd in Friesland. This village, built on a large mound, has a mysterious crypt (discovered by accident in 1765) in a small church dating from 1200. The corpses interred there centuries ago have never decomposed. One of the mummified bodies on display – that of the goldsmith Stellingwerf – has a virtually intact but completely leathery penis!

The penises of the dead can sometimes literally lead a life of their own. There are many stories in circulation about that of the deceased French emperor Napoleon – many and varied stories, comparable to the Arthurian legends. It is a historical fact that a post-mortem was carried out on the late emperor in 1821. It emerged that he had died of stomach cancer, quite a common occurrence in his family. The doctor conducting the post-mortem stated that the imperial reproductive

organs were small and insignificant and clearly shrivelled and desic-
cated. 'It should be pointed out, for the sake of historical truth, that the
deceased must have been completely impotent before his death.'

In his book P. Roobjee mentions that a priest who had been present
at the post-mortem somehow acquired Napoleon's penis and describes
what happened thereafter:

> It suddenly turned up again in the 1950s, after a mysterious
> odyssey of almost a hundred and fifty years, at Christie's Fine
> Art Auctioneers in London. The imperial member, one inch
> (2.54 cm) long, bore, according to a member of the staff who
> assisted at the sale, a strong resemblance to a very small sea-
> horse.

The auctioneer actually spoke of an insignificant, dried-up object.
There turned out to be no interest in the penis, on offer for £13,300.
Shortly afterwards the member was offered for sale in the catalogue of
a mail-order company, but again there were no takers. In 1961
Napoleon's penis finally acquired a worthy permanent owner, an
American urologist, who paid out approximately $3,800,000 for the
tiny object. Unfortunately the owner of the jewel was not able to enjoy
the sight of the Corsican-bred tufted-gilled seahorse for very long,
succumbing shortly afterwards to thrombosis and embolism of the
lung. Since then the member has begun a second secret odyssey and to
this day Napoleon's body lies – minus a penis – in the crypt beneath the
Dôme des Invalides.

The average length of the erect male penis is approximately five times
greater than that of an adult gorilla. Man's proportionately huge penis
gives an indirect indication of the sex lives of our forefathers. If we
bring evolution into the picture, a relatively long penis may have been
intended to scare off other males. While this is true of a few species of
monkeys, it probably doesn't work like that in man. Or is a long penis
intended to lure women? To heighten sexual pleasure? Neither of those
possibilities seems probable.

Evolutionary biologists argue that in the case of females who mate
with several males, the male with the longest penis delivers his sperm
cells most safely, and in other words has the best chance of fathering
progeny. Therefore the so-called sperm competition theory offers the
most elegant explanation of the dimensions of the penis. The vagina
is, believe it or not, a dreadful place for the sperm cell, an acidic torture chamber, which is why a penis that can reach the back of the
vagina has an advantage over one that delivers its content less close to

the ovum. Male seminal fluid is fortunately sufficiently alkaline to neutralize the acid. Because it is an advantage if a large quantity of sperm cells can be delivered close to the ova, in terms of evolutionary biology a condition has been created to make the penis grow in length. But a penis that reaches further than the mouth of the uterus no longer offers any extra advantage.

Koro

A very specific form of impotence, called *koro*, occurs in China and South-East Asia. The word is of Malay origin and means the head of a tortoise. It describes a psychiatric syndrome, in which the usually older patient becomes convinced that his penis is shrinking and will disappear into his abdomen (like a tortoise's head), finally resulting in death. *Koro* may be an expression of schizophrenia, a serious depression, epilepsy, a delirium, but may also occur in withdrawal from heroin, and very occasionally is the result of a brain tumour.

The Chinese term for the phenomenon is *suo-yang*, which means 'shrivelling penis'. There are various explanations for the fact that *koro* apparently occurs mainly in China. One of these is connected with Chinese philosophy and its yin–yang principle. According to this philo-sophy, man, the world and the cosmos are assigned two fundamental forces. Yang stands for hardness, firmness, the heavens, light, god, truth, drought, the left-hand and front side, and masculinity. Yin stands for the earth, calm, softness, the moon, darkness, deceitfulness, liquid, the right-hand and rear side, and femininity. For the man this means that both a drastic loss of yang and an excess of yin can lead to prob-lems. According to this view nocturnal emissions and masturbation cause a loss of yang. Normal coitus, between man and woman, that is, results in a 'healthy' exchange of yin and yang fluids.

More than in other cultures extensive use is made in China of potency-enhancing medicines. Quite understandable if one knows that male potency is directly related to the cosmic characteristics of the yang principle.

Koro also occurs in Western culture. In 1985 an article appeared in the *International Journal of Social Psychiatry* about an American patient in his fifties. He had reported to an emergency clinic with extreme anxiety, palpitations and hyperventilation. Shortly before he had visited a prostitute, who before giving him oral sex had washed his glans and penis – according to the patient – with a strange chemi-cal substance. Immediately afterwards, he claimed, his penis had started to shrivel. He had seen a strange smile on her face, and felt as if he were under a spell. It emerged that he was afraid of dying suddenly. He was admitted, after which it gradually became clear that he followed a solitary, schizoid lifestyle, and also drank far too heavily. Such stories were recorded in Europe too as far back as the fifteenth century, though not by psychiatrists, but by notorious witch-hunters. As is almost always the case, it is the woman who was demonized!

Misunderstandings about the glans

First, a few misunderstandings need clearing up: one, that the penis is a highly sensitive organ. That is totally untrue: the number of free nerve endings, compared, for example, with the lips, is extremely small. Only underneath the glans are there a relatively large number of free nerve endings.

The second misunderstanding is that the penis has to be active to become erect. This is also untrue: on the contrary, in order for the penis to stay flaccid the smooth muscle cells in the erectile tissue of the penis are contracted virtually all day long. At night during the REM sleep phase, and in sexual arousal, these smooth muscle cells relax, the spongiform network in the erectile tissue can enlarge and there is an erection.

The third, most serious misunderstanding is that the sole purpose of the glans or head of the penis is to be sucked on. It's true that the glans is soft, but for a quite different reason. In the view of the gynaecologist Robert Latou Dickinson (1861–1950) it had become soft in the course of evolution so as not to put too much pressure on the woman's internal sex organs during intercourse. However, this proved an incorrect interpretation.

The glans forms the end of the *corpus spongiosum*, the mass of erectile tissue surrounding the urethra. Just as in the twin sections of erectile tissue, the *corpora cavernosa,* the pressure in the corpus spongiosum increases during erection, but to a much lesser extent than in the corpora cavernosa. Otherwise the urethra would be squeezed shut so that the sperm could not be discharged at its intended destination.

Relatively little attention has been paid to the glans in poetry. Only the short-lived, doomed, alcoholic poet Paul Verlaine sang its praises in 'Hombres' (1891): 'my choice morsel, with its gush of divine phosphorus'. The poem is part of a collection published clandestinely after his death, in which this famous poet presents himself licking and gorging, revelling in sex with women, but also yearning for homosexual love.

In Ancient Greece competitors in the Olympic Games were naked. However, it was forbidden for them to display their glans – that was considered vulgar. So a ribbon was bound round the foreskin, for what reason is not entirely clear.

Compression
of exiting blood
vessels in erection

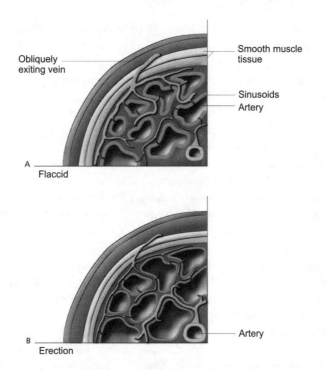

Obliquely
exiting vein

Smooth muscle
tissue

Sinusoids
Artery

A

Flaccid

B

Erection

Artery

In ruminants a globe-shaped glans transforms into a thread-like appendage, which during mating extends into the uterus; in rams this is 4 cm long. In carnivores and insectivores there are spines and thorns in the glans. At rest these are hidden in a kind of sac. In an erection, however, they protrude, giving the female extra stimulation. Such protuberances occur in man too. In the scientific literature there are descriptions of almost a hundred patients with such abnormalities. They are almost always a kind of horn, which in over 30 per cent of cases involves cancer. Treatment is fortunately simple and usually solves the problem: the diseased part is removed surgically. Urologists call this a partial penis amputation, though after such a disfiguring operation it is still perfectly possible to enjoy a normal sex life. Unfortunately there is often a lack of good counselling in such cases.

In certain cultures men made protrusions for their glans. In nine-teenth-century Java, for example, this was quite normal. Grooves were cut in several places and filled with tiny stones. Once the wounds were completely healed, the glans had an irregular, bumpy surface which provided extra vaginal stimulation. For the same purpose the Dayaks and other primitive peoples drove a bamboo pipe right through the glans or put a bone through it. When performing everyday activities the bone was replaced by a feather; only the tribal chief was entitled to have a second hole made. In Europe too people looked for ways to increase women's pleasure in coitus. In eighteenth-century France penis rings with hard protuberances, called *aides*, were used, while in Russia such rings were fitted with tiny white teeth; in South America the preference was for horsehair. Modern ribbed condoms are the latest variant.

The genitalia of the kamikaze drone of the honey bee are also decorated, with yellowish protuberances and all kinds of fringes and hairs: at orgasm they explode within the queen like a spring and form a natural chastity belt, which bars access to other suitors, even though the mating drone itself drops dead.

Some rodents and felines are blessed with true foreskin glands, producing, for example, musk, which quite a few women use in perfume on a daily basis. (Assuming that perfumes are intended to attract men, it is odd that women should use male glandular secretions.) It is true that Homo sapiens also has glands near the foreskin, but they are usually a source of great worry and misery. Countless patients think they have contracted a venereal disease when they first observe the sebaceous glands on the underside of the head of their penis. In yet another category of patients, not used to pulling back the foreskin on a daily basis and washing the glans, abundant sebaceous secretions accumulate beneath the foreskin. These are called smegma, a whitish substance with the consistency of bath soap, which accumulates in the folds of the sex organs. In the view of some scientists smegma is carcinogenic. To put it more delicately, it is soap that does not cleanse. Before a urologist can examine the inside of the bladder, the penis must first be disinfected. This places quite a burden on nursing staff, who have to disinfect up to fifteen penises a day. One nurse in my department refers to these sebaceous secretions as 'home-made cheese'.

Going hard, going soft

In only a few men (a mere 8%) is the erect penis completely vertical. In between 15 and 20 per cent the angle of erection is approximately 45 per cent above horizontal, though on average it is above the horizontal. The penis is suspended on bands, in such a way that when erect it pulls towards the abdomen.

The fact that the male penis is so prominently visible may explain why nude photos of women were accepted much earlier than those of men. Because of the need to point when urinating, boys become acquainted with their penis at an early age, and hence it comes as no surprise that boys start masturbating at a younger age than girls. In the course of time, while cycling or horse-riding, they notice that stimulation of the penis can produce a pleasant sensation. Quite a few young

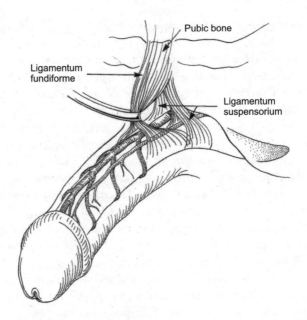

The suspension bands.

men worry about what they regard as a lopsided penis, which they blame on excessive masturbation. Their concern is completely groundless. Every man's penis is slightly askew, as mentioned previously, usually inclining towards the left. On the basis of interviews the American researcher Alfred Kinsey (1894–1956) claimed as long ago as the 1950s that between 70 and 80 per cent of men hang to the left. This was confirmed – incredibly – after scientific research by radiologists. It was noted how the penis hung on a large series of x-ray photos of the pelvis minor. The point is that on a blank x-ray, that is, one without contrast, the penis is easily visible as 'soft-tissue shadow', as it is called in medical jargon.

Certainly, there is increasing interest in sexology in radiodiagnostics. In fact, the first magnetic resonance imaging of coitus was carried out in Groningen in the 1990s. This requires a couple to make love to order in the narrow tunnel of an MRI scanner. It is scarcely surprising that many male test subjects were unable to perform. Women of course did not experience the same problem. In addition, this research showed that the penis penetrates less far into the woman's body than doctors had hitherto assumed.

The penis is nothing but a big blood sausage, albeit one consisting of three compartments, or masses of spongiform erectile tissue. When it is engorged with blood as a result of sexual arousal and there is very little drainage, the penis becomes hard and stiff, and an erection occurs. The twin erectile tissue compartments on the top of the penis, the *corpora cavernosa*, fill first, followed by the third compartment, the *corpus spongiosum*. The two upper compartments are linked in several places, and their ends are attached to the underside of the pubic bone. At the top the previously mentioned suspension bands act as a kind of lever between these erectile tissue compartments and the upper surface of the pubic bone. Otherwise the erect penis would start flopping about. The third compartment surrounds the urethra and runs into the glans. Surrounding the head is the foreskin, which can easily slide back. Unlike the shaft of the penis, the glans is reasonably well equipped with nerve endings, of which the *frenulum* or 'little bridle' is the most sensitive. Under the skin of the pelvis, besides a thin layer of connective tissue, there is a sturdy sheet of the same tissue. This sheet is adjacent to the casing of the erectile tissue compartments, the *tunica albuginea*.

Since the erection is brought about by vasocongestion in the erectile tissue compartments, it is important that the relevant arteries are intact. These are in order: the great abdominal aorta, which divides into two in the pelvis, and branches of which go to the leg, the buttock and the penis. The two arteries leading to the penis each have three branches: one runs across the top of the penis, one through the middle of the *corpora cavernosa* and one through the *corpus spongiosum*. Those running through the two *corpora cavernosa* are the most important: they branch into countless tiny arteries and join the tiny veins that drain the blood off again. These small veins discharge into larger veins in the erectile tissue compartments that subsequently drain the blood into the inferior caval vein in the abdomen.

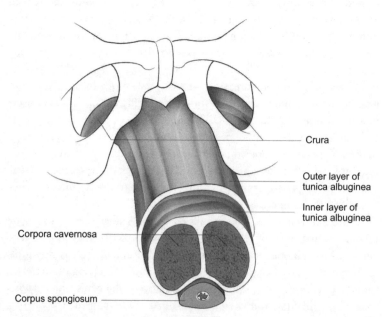

Crura

Outer layer of
tunica albuginea

Inner layer of
tunica albuginea

Corpora cavernosa

Corpus spongiosum

Cross-section of
the penis and the
pubic bone.

The blood supply
to the penis.

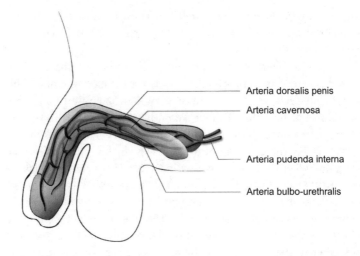

Arteria dorsalis penis

Arteria cavernosa

Arteria pudenda interna

Arteria bulbo-urethralis

In order to produce an erection the veins must widen, the muscles on the spongiform tissue in the compartments must relax, and the veins must be somewhat compressed. This happens through the effect of nervous stimuli. There are two erection centres in the spine for this purpose, one level with the sacrum and one with the lumbar vertebrae. If, for example, there is complete paralysis of the lower body as a result of a spinal fracture, an erection may still be produced through manual stimulation, a so-called reflex erection. As soon as the stimulation stops, the erection disappears. Coitus is not possible.

Is the penis actually eatable as a blood sausage? Yes: Midas Dekkers writes about this in his book on bestiality, *Dearest Pet*. The recipe comes from the humble Jewish Yemeni culinary tradition: blanch and clean a goat's penis. Boil for ten minutes and cut into slices. Sauté onions, garlic and coriander in oil. Add the penis and fry. Mix chopped tomatoes, pepper, cumin, saffron and salt and pour the mixture over the penis. Cover the pan and braise slowly for two hours until cooked. Experts have found the taste disappointing.

The vagina dentata

Some men are incapable of giving themselves sexually. They act tough, but really they're wimps: their penis goes limp when they try to man-oeuvre it into the vagina. This is not true impotence, but is caused by the deep-seated fear of losing their beloved organ, fear of the *vagina dentata*, the sharp-toothed vagina, with which a man's penis can be bitten off. The vagina dentata plays an important part in an old African legend: beautiful girls descend to earth from heaven and repeatedly steal a hunter's bag. When a man keeping guard catches them, he shoots one of them, but pays for his attempt to rape her with his member: her vagina contains extremely sharp teeth, with which she bites off his penis.

An age-old Siberian fairy tale also tells of the vagina dentata, though this story has a fairly happy ending for the man. On one of his journeys a hunter meets a one-eyed cave-dweller. She claims him as her husband, but he hesitates. Though he finds her big breasts appealing, her strange face deters him. There is also a sound emanating from her body that is like the gnashing of teeth. When she has fallen asleep, he investigates where the noise is coming from. Between her legs he discovers two rows of teeth. The hunter then devises a trick. He looks for an oblong stone and when the woman wakes up and wants sex with him he puts the stone between his legs and her secret teeth grind and break on the rock-hard material until her vagina becomes like that of any other woman. Eventually the man takes her home with him as his slave.

The vagina dentata is also found in modern feminist literature. Ela, the heroine of the novel *F/32*, the debut of the Greek writer Eurydice Kamvisseli, has an amazingly tight and greedy sex organ, which is inexhaustibly described. She has a fan club of hundreds of ex-lovers, who wear a coloured ribbon round their penis, marking their place in the strict hierarchy of sexual feats. The book contains unforgettably amusing, instructive and enchanting passages. This is one from the prologue:

> Ela presents her cunt to men with great abandon, as if it were John the Baptist's silver-tongued head on a platter, gives them license to do anything to it, to try their luck and not spare it . . . 'Don't mistake my cunt for the *kudos*,' Ela warns men at times, hoping to tip the scales . . . 'Enter it at your own risk.' They break into a cocky laugh.

Not long afterwards her cunt devours them whole . . . If you didn't know, it must be clear by now. The fear of the vagina dentata and the accompanying premature loss of erection before entering, are as old as mankind. The only thing that helps is to talk about it.

Men obviously sometimes have weird ideas about female genitalia: not only that there are teeth set in them, but also that women have two vaginas rather than one. This is an age-old theme described by the Italian Poggio Bracciolini in his fifteenth-century *Liber facetiarum* (Book of Humour): a completely idiotic farmer, who hasn't a clue about sex, gets married. In bed he thrusts his 'spear' into his wife's backside. Delighted at his successful attempt he asks her if by any chance she has two vaginas: one is enough for him, the second is superfluous. The wife, who is having an affair with the parish priest, then proposes donating her second one to the church. The farmer of course agrees. The couple invite the priest to supper, and after the meal they all get into bed. The priest first introduces his member and the stupid farmer makes do with his portion. 'Remember our agreement, use your own share and leave mine to me,' says the farmer. To which the priest replies: 'As God is my witness: I don't desire your portion in the least, as long as I may use the church's share.' The priest can carry on as before.

Doctors used to link the size of the nose and the dimensions of the genitalia. The idea was shown to be absurd, but there *are* so-called *nasogenital alliances*. One of these is the anatomical affinity between the erectile tissue compartments in the penis and those in the clitoris and the olfactory mucous membrane. When someone becomes sexually aroused, the olfactory mucous membrane tends to become rather swollen. As a result sexually stimulated people have slightly more difficulty in breathing through their nose. It can happen that a man has the urge to sneeze when confronted with an attractive woman. There is obviously after all a link between the nose and the sex organs. No wonder that in Ancient Rome adulterous men had not their penis, but their nose cut off!

There are complicated forms of cooperation between the sense of smell, the sex hormones and the sexual urge. These operate through pheromones. The word 'pheromone' is a contraction of the Greek words *fero* (transfer/carry) and *hormao* (set in motion). Pheromones are substances that secrete organisms in order to induce a reaction in members of the same species. They do this through various glands. A male pig, for example, produces the pheromone androstenol in its mouth which causes a fertile sow to go rigid, so that he can mount her at his leisure.

Pheromones can be picked up via the tastebuds and olfactory receptors, on the tongue, in the nose or via Jacobson's organ. The latter is situated on the floor of the nasal cavities of, for example, reptiles and mammals. In man it has become rudimentary in the course of evolution; researchers from the University of Michigan recently showed that the two genes that govern signal transfer in Jacobson's organ are no longer functional in man or anthropoid apes. The genes are there but 22 million years ago were shifted to an inactive chromosome section. The loss of pheromonal communication was compensated for by the gradually acquired ability to see a wider colour spectrum (red, orange and green).

Length

From an early age one hears the complaint, sometimes disguised, about being under-endowed. According to the American sexologist Barry McCarthy, two out of three men think their penis is too small. He attributes their worries about the length of their penises to various factors.

In the first place little boys see their father's penis for the first time when they are at an impressionable age. Second, in changing rooms one usually sees another person's penis from the front: the other person's penis appears to be bigger because a man can only see his own penis from above. Seen from above, however, there is what visual artists call 'foreshortening'. The penis seems smaller than it really is. Third, flaccid penises can differ widely in length, while in erect ones on the other hand there is never that much difference. And fourth, men don't know much about the subject in general, because they don't like talking openly about these kinds of intimate matters.

The problem of penis length is as old as the hills: in eighteenth-century Normandy it was for that reason customary for midwives to keep the umbilical cords of male babies relatively long. If the cord was pulled too tight in tying it and was therefore cut off too short, the member would be pulled inside.

In 1899 the German doctor Loeb carried out research with fifty men between eighteen and 53: the length of the visible part of the flaccid penis varied from 8 to 11 cm (average 9.4 cm) and the circumference from 8 to over 10 cm. It emerged from the Kinsey Report that only a quarter of men have an erect penis of 'average' size. But extremes are rare: 5 per cent of men have an erection of less than 9 cm and only 1 per cent can boast a massive erection of over 20 cm.

Doctor Jacobus X was the pseudonym of a surgeon in the French army who devoted years of his life to examining and measuring hundreds of sex organs of men and women from all over the world. Comparative research was his passion. In 1935 he published the results of his work, which showed that black Africans had the longest penises, varying when flaccid from 12 to 15 cm, and erect from 19 to 29 cm. Jacobus observes that penis size is always commensurate with vagina size in the same race. 'Hindustani women, whose men have slim, short penises, will have difficulty in accommodating the average European,' wrote the army doctor, 'and in their eyes the huge penis of a black African would be an instrument of torture.'

Jacobus appears to be saying that nature ensures that people of the same race seek each other out. From this perspective mixing of the races is unnatural. Nowadays we would frown at such views but in the 1930s such notions were not uncommon.

Peno-scrotal
webbing

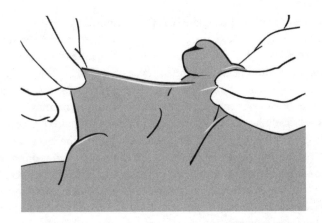

However, Piesol's manual of anatomy (1907) already states that in comparison with other organs penis size is not connected with physical development. You cannot tell the length of a man's penis from his nose, as some mothers-in-law occasionally maintain. There is, though, according to the scientists Siminoski and Bain, a statistically significant correlation between a man's shoe size and the length of his penis.

A particular form of small penis is the *penis palmatus*. In this case the penis is not in fact too small, but appears to be so because the penis and the skin of the scrotum have as it were grown together to form a kind of web. It is usually sufficient to cut the web across and reattach it lengthways.

Occasionally even politicians become involved with stiff penises. In 1993 a debate developed in the European Parliament on penis length. A Dutch Green MP asked the Commission to put an end to 'the squabbling about EU norms for condoms'. What was the problem? There had to be European norms for everything under the sun. The British argued for a compromise on the length and diameter of the European penis. In their view an average erect length of 17 cm and 5.6 cm diameter was a gross underestimate. The average British penis, they maintained, was considerably larger. The Dutch MEP asked the Commission if it did not agree that, in view of obvious sensitivities that existed regarding the establishment of the average length of the sexual organ, it would be sensible simply to allow each country to maintain its own average, or in any case to debate it at a level below the European one. She saw a European charter for the condom as an alternative possibility. Member states could then argue for exceptions to the statistically estimated average. 'And if the gentlemen simply can't crack the problem, perhaps the male member itself should be standardized, I'm curious to know what the regulation wonks in Brussels would come up with,' concluded the MEP.

The psychologist Erick Janssen was commissioned by the Amsterdam condom store The Golden Fleece to investigate the circumference of the erect penis. If a condom is too tight, it can lead to complaints, ranging from 'doesn't fit' to 'chokes everything off', while a condom that is too loose can of course slide off prematurely. He found that the average diameter of the fully erect penis was approximately 121 mm, with a relatively large spread, from 90 to 161 mm. It also emerged that in a quarter of the test subjects the circumference of the erect penis was less than 110 mm, in three-quarters less than 130 mm and in 90 per cent less than 140 mm. In 10 per cent the circumference of the erect penis was over 140 mm. The researcher's conclusion was that good consumer advice on condoms should always contain information on penis thicknesses in relation to various sizes of condom.

In ancient Tantric texts the length of the penis is measured from the perineum, that is, from beneath the testicles. Measured in this way penises of up to 30 cm are quite normal. Perhaps we Westerners are selling ourselves short, and perhaps it feels 'fuller and more whole' if you include the testicles as well.

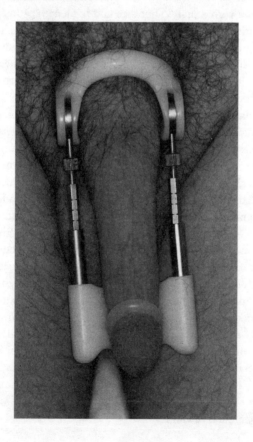

The JES extender.

Lengthening

Down the ages men have tried to make their penises longer. The most primitive method is to hang stones from it. This does work, but also causes impotence. Then there was the Polynesian stretching method using a movable weighted tube, the Arab *jelq* treatment (massage), and the penicure based on it: in the United States there are apparatuses on sale that massage according to the *jelq* method. The supplier claims that a lengthening of 2.5 cm can be achieved within twenty weeks. Full details are to be found in Gary Griffith's *Penis Enlargement Methods*.

According to Jolan Chang, author of *The Tao of Love and Sex,* the most important thing is practice, since Taoists believe that absolutely every part of the human body can be trained and developed. The Chinese did after all invent physiotherapy!

In the summer of 1993 the under-endowed were pleasantly surprised by reports in the gay press that over a hundred penis-lengthening operations had been carried out in South Africa. When questioned, the Johannesburg-based plastic surgeon responsible stated that the patient 'resumes his normal sex life after a month. He has only a small scar that extends down to the scrotum. The patient achieves an incredible result with very little discomfort.' According to the same report it would not be very long before similar surgery was introduced into Europe.

Well, in August 1994 the moment arrived. A urologist from Utrecht announced in an interview with a leading daily that *he* had attempted the experimental operation. 'It's a simple procedure, we took over two hours, at a leisurely pace, but it's possible to do it in an hour and a half. It really gives a very nice result. The patient thought so too. He just can't get enough of looking under the covers. I'm his hero,' said the urologist. The report, partly because of the unfortunate choice of words by the otherwise media-friendly urologist, caused a great uproar: the hospital director, a university expert on andrology, a celebrated plastic surgeon, board members of the Dutch Association of Urology, a medical ethics specialist and a gay newspaper editor, all had their say in the daily press.

With the exception of the last three all expressed serious misgivings. The andrologist worried about anatomical proportions: 'The question is whether this can be done with impunity, since it changes the suspension of the penis. Is that possible? It could snap,' said the professor. The hospital director and the medical ethicist were in total agreement: 'In future a medical ethics committee must first be consulted.' The poor urologist didn't really understand the resistance. 'For the moment there is no reason to reject penis-lengthening. The only publications on the subject are in Chinese, so let me first do some research, carry out a series of operations and publish the results.'

Unfortunately, it is clear that neither the urologist in question, nor any of the commentators knew the scientific literature. The operation performed turns out to be nothing but a variant of one that has been known about for years, and which is in fact in no way experimental. The essence of the procedure is that the band by which the penis is attached to the pubic bone at the front (the *ligamentum suspensorium*) is severed. In this way the 'hanging portion' of the penis is lengthened. At the same time the operating surgeon makes the incision in such a way that the skin too can be slid towards the penis. He/she stitches the skin in a different direction from that of the incision. In the jargon it is called Y-V or double Z cosmetic surgery.

Incidentally, there are also techniques for thickening the penis, but that is a completely different story. One method is to transplant subcutaneous fat tissue. The results are mediocre and aftercare is problematic, but large sums of money are involved in it.

Experts – child urologists and urologists with a sexological orientation – have long been in agreement: in men with a penis length of under 4 cm there may be good reason, partly on the advice of a sexologist, to decide on a penis-lengthening procedure. By way of comparison: the average length of the penis in newborn infants is 3.5 cm. Since 1975 penis experts have been able to use the scientifically based table overleaf, giving normal penis dimensions. Little is known about the causes of an undersized penis. Possibly a deficiency in male sex hormone in the final stages of pregnancy is involved. The abnormality may

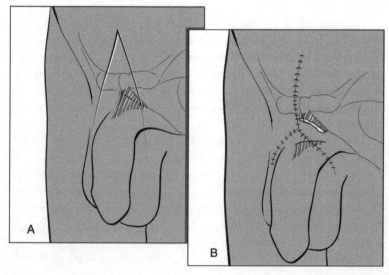

Penis lengthening surgery.

be found in isolation, but may also be part of innate anatomical and endocrinological conditions.

Before deciding on an operation for penis lengthening there should always be a consultation, preferably with an expert sexologist. The following facts should be remembered:

The smaller the penis, the bigger the erection will be in proportion.

It is only friction in the outermost portion of the vagina that counts.

The vagina adjusts to every size of penis.

Dutch women consider circumference more important than length.

It's not what you've got, it's what you do with it.

There's always someone worse off than you are!

Age	Average approx. SD* cm	Average -2.5 SD cm
Infant 30 weeks	2.5 approx. 0.4	1.5 cm
Infant 40 weeks	3.0 approx. 0.4	2.0 cm
Infant full-term	3.5 approx. 0.4	2.4 cm
0–15 months	3.9 approx. 0.8	1.9 cm
6–12 months	4.3 approx. 0.8	2.3 cm
1–2 years	4.7 approx. 0.8	2.6 cm
2–3 years	5.1 approx. 0.9	2.9 cm
3–4 years	5.5 approx. 0.9	3.3 cm
4–5 years	5.7 approx. 0.9	3.5 cm
5–6 years	6.0 approx. 0.9	3.7 cm
6–7 years	6.1 approx. 0.9	3.8 cm
7–8 years	6.2 approx. 1.0	3.7 cm
8–9 years	6.3 approx. 1.0	3.8 cm
9–10 years	6.3 approx. 1.0	3.8 cm
10–11 years	6.4 approx. 1.1	3.7 cm
Adults	13.3 approx. 1.6	9.3 cm

Table: Penis Length in Normal Men.
*SD = standard deviation

Source: K. W. Feldman and D. W. Smith, 'Fetal phallic growth and penile standards for new born male infants', *Journal of Pediatrics*, 86 (1975), p. 395.

With these rules in mind the great majority of men can overcome their worries about the length of their penis! Apart from that there are some practical tips one can give: don't wear jeans or briefs – Bermudas or boxer shorts are better – and trim over-abundant pubic hair.

If the patient continues to fret, the results of the scientific research carried out by psychologist William A. Fisher should be discussed. He attempted to measure the effect of penis size on the degree of sexual arousal in both women and men (students). In stories about love-making the penis either was not mentioned (control condition) or *was* mentioned (experimental condition). In the description of the penis the length was mentioned five times per story. The length varied from story to story as follows: small – 7.5 cm, average – 12.5 cm, large – 20 cm. After reading a story the test subjects assessed their own level of arousal and had to indicate how aroused the man and woman in the story were. When asked afterwards about their memory of the content of the story the control group quite rightly did not mention the length of the penis. The experimental group did, especially the group that read the description of the large penis. No difference was observed between men and women. So the test subjects had noticed the nature of the description. However, the test subjects could not afterwards indicate what the point of the research was. Yet the observed length of the penis turned out to contribute nothing to the subjects' assessment of their own degree of arousal. 'Variation in the length of the penis therefore does nor appear to be a precondition for arousal,' the authors of the article conclude.

The American psychologist Bernie Zilbergeld has incidentally pointed out that men with a relatively large penis can become impotent because, for instance, of the fear that they will hurt their partner during intercourse, or the fact that they were rejected at some time in the past because of their large penis.

In a 1994 article in a gay newspaper entitled 'Willies. On Genitalia', Cees van der Pluijm cites a 1967 study by an interestingly named American scientist called Havelock Eliott. The latter's *On Penises* (1967), purportedly includes numerous interesting facts about size and particularly about the correlation between size and other characteristics. It emerges that athletes had on average not only a longer, but also a significantly thicker penis. In over 80 per cent of swimmers the penis was shown to be small.

Eliott is also reported, somewhat less plausibly, as having investigated the relationship between penis length and political affiliation. Republicans score significantly higher than Democrats, while the most conservative Republicans are in turn among the best-hung individuals in their party. The hypothesis that men with left-wing sympathies are often below par, we are told, proves in 69.8 per cent of cases to have a basis in truth, though the suggestion that changing one's voting behaviour might affect the penis length is dismissed by the researcher. If true, these would be sensational findings, but the absence of the book in question from every major library catalogue consulted confirms one's growing suspicion that Van der Pluijm's piece is a sophisticated spoof.

chapter three

The Prostate and Seminal Glands

Some women have endless trouble with their womb: for decades they endure the discomfort of painful periods, and then, just as hormonal retirement beckons, on come the hot flushes, to say nothing of other afflictions. Women sometimes feel that life has been unfair to them in this respect; that isn't so. Men have their own cross to bear, namely the prostate, a gland that only receives proper attention when it starts playing up. Then the prostrate becomes a bane, not only keeping a man awake at night, but also inconveniencing him in everyday activities like

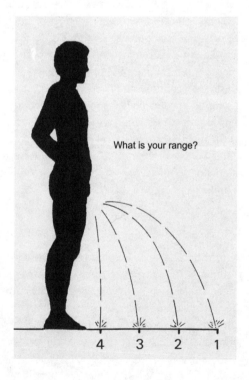

Men's troubles.

going to meetings. Urinating becomes a depressing business. Men's troubles! The prostate is thoroughly out of favour nowadays. Many women have children with the aid of test tubes, pipettes and incubators, and no longer have any need for it . . .

So is the prostate perhaps not that important after all? For example, there has never yet been a prostate transplant. There is no country on earth where the prostate is eaten, in contrast to testes (for example, in Spain) and penis (as blood sausage in Yemen). Odd, when one knows that in operations to resection the prostate via the urethra urologists fish out what look like strips of kebab.

Historically, the prostate came into its own at a quite late stage. Prostate problems were unknown in Ancient Egypt, undoubtedly partly because people did not live as long as they do now. Similarly, Hippocrates ($c.$460–$c.$370 BC) writes nothing about the subject. The term was first used by Herophilus, who several centuries before Christ founded the famous school of Alexandria. Even Rudolf Virchow, the founder of modern pathology, collected only a few prostates in formalin.

Anatomy and physiology

Only a small percentage of the total volume of an ejaculate is made up of sperm cells. In older medical literature, as previously mentioned, a distinction was made between the sperm-cell portion or 'nobler part', 'the aqueous elements' from the seminal glands and the 'oleagenous' portion from the prostate. The prostate is about the size of a chestnut. The seminal glands are situated behind it and discharge into the urethra, which passes right through the prostate.

In animals the system is different. Dogs, like many other carnivores, have very small seminal glands. The reason why is a complete mystery. In man the fluid produced by the seminal glands is important mainly for the mobility and the metabolism of sperm cells. In humans it can make up between 50 and 80 per cent of the total volume of ejaculate. The principal ingredients of seminal fluid are fructose, coagulating agents and the prostaglandins E, A, D and F.

The finger in the anus

For years the significance of the so-called rectal toucher (RT) in relation to urinary ailments has been controversial. In this procedure the doctor puts a finger up the anus and feels the prostate and the mucous membrane of the rectum. The gravity of urinary complaints is rarely if ever related to the size of the prostate, whether this is assessed with the finger or by using ultrasound. In fact the size of the prostate is only of

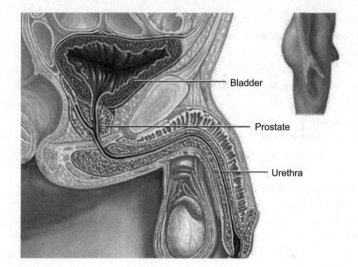

Bladder

Prostate

Urethra

Anatomy of the prostate and the urethra.

importance to the urologist in deciding on the type of operation recommended, via the urethra or via an incision in the abdomen. Estimating the size of the prostate using RT depends undeniably on the experience of the person carrying out the examination. In general the size of a large prostate tends to be underestimated and that of a small one overestimated in RT. The assessment of consistency can provide an indication as to whether there is a benign enlargement, an inflammation or a cancer. The benign prostate has the consistency of the ball of a closed fist, cancer feels as hard as the joint between the metacarpals and the first phalanx bone in the hand, and in the case of inflammation the prostate feels as soft as the ball of the thumb with the fingers spread.

With RT the feelings of both the person examining and the patient are much more involved than in a general physical examination. It is not inconceivable that certain emotional reactions may lead to RT being skipped altogether. Research in the UK showed that with almost two-thirds of patients with urinary complaints GPs omitted to carry out RT before referral. In addition it is well known that insufficient training of medical students leads to postponement and avoidance behaviour in later professional life. Nowadays, in many medical faculties there are systematic skills training courses in preparation for later practice. In a number of faculties specially trained instructors are used.

Benign prostate enlargement

A chronically enlarged prostate can lead to bladder stones, in the past much more frequently than now. The great religious reformer Calvin was a sufferer. 'When he could no longer endure the pain,' writes the

Italian essayist Guido Ceronetti, 'the old Calvin [in 1563 he was 54, which in those days counted as old] mounted his horse on his doctors' advice, and rode at the trot, in dreadful pain, until the jolting caused the stone to descend into the urethra.' On returning home he urinated slimy blood and the following day the stone – as big as a hazelnut – was expelled with the aid of hot compresses. This was followed by a spurt of blood. 'Thus God relieved Calvin of the stone and left the stone, with Calvin, to the inhabitants of Geneva,' wrote Ceronetti.

Bladder stones and incontinence are only two in a whole spectrum of prostate ailments. Other problems caused by an obstructive prostate are urinary blockage, or the inability to urinate, renal pelvic inflammation and loss of the kidneys. Fortunately things rarely if ever reach that stage nowadays. More frequent urination, a less powerful stream of urine, dribbling and suchlike prompt men to consult their GP in good time. The taboo surrounding prostate ailments has gone. The worried well with minor problems often need no treatment, rather reassurance about the presence or otherwise of prostate cancer. With moderate symptoms it is preferable to start with medication. Only if that fails to solve the problem is there reason to consult a urologist, who may choose to operate in one of two ways: via the urethra or, if the prostate is very enlarged, via an abdominal incision. Complications include incontinence, in most cases temporary, narrowing of the urethra (5% risk), and blood loss in the urine, sometimes continuing for a period of weeks. Up to now alternative treatments such as warming the prostate ('microwave' therapy) have proved less effective.

Blood in sperm

In order to understand the sexual experiences of his or her fellow-humans a urologist must be a man or woman of the world: broadminded and with sufficient powers of imagination. Even when you think you possess these qualities, you can occasionally come across a case like the following, which remains baffling.

A 50-year-old homosexual man comes to the outpatient clinic complaining that his sperm 'is always coloured'. 'Haemospermia' is my immediate thought. He had been examined two days before and nothing abnormal had been found. 'Reassured patient,' said the notes, but had that really reassured him? 'So all that time there was blood in your sperm?' 'Yes, every time, sometimes red, sometimes brown or yellow, sometimes with lumps or streaks, and sometimes watery.' The patient tells me this with some distaste, but in great detail, which many men would find impossible. Repeated examinations reveal no abnormalities. 'You're not doing anything . . .' I ask hesitantly. 'Nothing special, just hand-jobs, together,' replies the patient. 'I should say I haven't got a permanent relationship, but when I pick someone up in the pub in the evenings and I come it's a real turn-off to keep seeing my sperm like that. It's really embarrassing. Or am I supposed to do it in the dark from now on?' 'Blood in sperm' can definitely spoil someone's love life, but the problem remains that in the vast majority of cases urological examinations relating to haemospermia reveal no abnormalities.

Inflammation of the prostate

'As men grow older they believe they still have abundant sexual energy, but they are being fooled by the signals they are receiving because these are being sent to them only by an irritated, worn-out prostate,' is how the Italian poet, philosopher, essayist and philosopher of science Guido Ceronetti characterized one of the problems of men suffering from inflammation of the prostate. Prostatitis is very common, more so in its chronic than in its acute form. Acute inflammation of the prostate is generally caused by a bacterium that penetrates the prostate from the urinary tract. This can happen easily since the prostate with its many drainage routes is directly linked to the urethra. Prostatitis is not always the result of a urinary tract infection – micro-organisms can also infect the prostate via the blood. Then there are venereal diseases, euphemistically called sexually transmitted diseases, which may lead to inflammations. In the past the main culprit was the clap, a gonoccochal infection; nowadays it is mostly chlamydia trachomatis. An added problem is that many women carry this micro-organism without being aware of it and so form a source of infection.

In cases of acute prostatitis the patient is unwell, has a high temperature and, because of swelling, urinating is painful and sometimes completely impossible. Treatment with an antibiotic that penetrates the prostate effectively can prevent the condition from worsening. In the worst-case scenario an abcess develops, which has to be drained by a urologist, usually through the rectum. With a chronic prostate infection things go on simmering: medication brings temporary relief, but after a while the symptoms return. Back pain, pain in the area between the scrotum and the anus (the feeling of sitting on a hot chestnut), a burning feeling when urinating, a frequent urge to urinate: these symptoms can drive sufferers to distraction. Sometimes the symptoms spill over into the patient's sexual functioning: there is a loss of sexual appetite, ejaculation becomes painful and in the worst case the man becomes impotent. Chronic prostate inflammation is sometimes the result of an inadequately treated acute inflammation. The bacteria hide in out-of-the-way corners and hence do not show up in urine cultures. A cure becomes difficult. In some cases stones, or accumulations of calcium, form in the prostate. Very occasionally long-term treatment with an antibiotic brings relief, but mostly it remains an ongoing problem.

Many men with prostatitis change doctors or ask for a second opinion, possibly because advice quite frequently differs widely: one doctor recommends hot baths, another cold ones, one urges less sex, the other . . . etc. That is understandable when one knows that the ailment does not follow a fixed pattern: sometimes the patient feels better after an ejaculation, sometimes even worse. What we do know is that alcohol never helps.

Prostate cancer

Prostate cancer is largely a disease of our age. Two centuries ago it was rare: patients died before the cancer manifested itself. The body is constantly under construction and in decomposition, cells die and are replaced by new ones. This constant renewal allows organs to function normally. If certain cells do not die and change in such a way that they start multiplying abnormally and develop into a malignant tumour, we speak of cancer. But there is huge variation within that diagnosis. These days many men are told that they have prostate cancer, but by no means all of them die of it, or if they do it is only much, much later.

A good example of this is the case history of former French president François Mitterrand (1916–1996). He was first diagnosed with prostate cancer in 1981 at the age of 65 and he died at the age of 79. Celebrated musician Frank Zappa (1940–1993) was unfortunately diagnosed too late, and died of the disease. The same happened to Prince Claus von Amsberg (1926–2000), husband of Queen Beatrix of the Netherlands, whose ordeal began with his diagnosis in 1998. He had an operation, but this was not radical enough, and subsequent microscopic examination showed that prostate cancer cells were still present, requiring a course of radiotherapy. A side-effect of the radiotherapy was that the draining of urine from the kidneys to the bladder became impeded, and hence one kidney had to be removed. The prince then developed intestinal problems that necessitated a colostomy, and from then on his condition went into a downward spiral, finally resulting in an embolism of the lung and a heart attack. In contrast, the Bond films actor Roger Moore was treated in time.

Mitterrand's experience shows that there is a form of prostate cancer that develops so slowly that it may be twenty years before the growth becomes life threatening. When such a process begins only at a late stage in life, at the age of 65, for example, the patient may experience some discomfort, but very frequently has no symptoms at all. With such a virtually benign form of prostate cancer one can live for years without any problem or symptom. Some urologists call these types of cancer 'pussycats', as opposed to the 'tigers', highly malignant and dangerous prostate cancers. Tigers can sometimes, but not always, be recognized by the pathologist by microscopic analysis when the diagnosis is made. The higher the Gleason sum score – named after the scientist who devised the best method of grading prostate cancer – the greater the chance that the cancer is a tiger.

In the spring of 1949 the philosopher Ludwig Wittgenstein felt more tired than usual and was found to be suffering from anaemia. At the end of the summer, on a visit to the United States, he became very ill and had to be admitted to hospital. He was not frightened of a diagnosis of a serious illness, but did dread an unnecessary prolonging of his life, leaving him to await death for years in a state of complete helplessness. What's more, he was frightened of dying in America and exclaimed to his host and ex-colleague Norman Malcolm: 'I don't want to die in America. I am a European. What a fool I was to come.' At first no sign of a serious disease was found, but back in England he was proved right. He wrote in a letter to Malcolm:

> I have prostate cancer. But it sounds much worse than it is, as there is medication which, so they tell me, may alleviate the symptoms of the disease, so that I may live for years yet. The doctor tells me that I may be able to work again, but I can't imagine that. I wasn't at all alarmed when I heard that I had cancer, but I was when they told me that they could treat me, because I have no desire to go on living. My wish was not granted. I'm being treated by everybody with the greatest kindness and I have a terribly kind doctor, who is no fool.

The man who wrote in his diary in 1930 'Very often or almost always I'm frightened to death', showed not a trace of fear when death approached.

For forty years Anatole Broyard was an editor, literary critic and essayist on the *New York Times*. At the age of 69 he was told that he had prostate cancer. He gives an account of this period in *Intoxicated by My Illness*, the main message of which is: 'I would advise every sick person to evolve a style or develop a voice for his or her illness. In my case I make fun of my illness.' Although the writer states that after hearing about his fatal disease he loses all belief in the irony of the human condition as such, he clings to his ironic perspective, which the diagnosis of cancer does not destroy. On his first visit to the specialist he takes a seat in the waiting room. Full of appreciation he studies the tasteful décor and counts himself fortunate that the doctor who designed this room is to be his doctor. The doctor comes in and asks Broyard to follow him to his room. He finds himself in a completely impersonal room with an equally impersonal consultant. He decides to change doctors: 'I found another urologist. He is brilliant, famous, a star and my response to him was so positive that my cancer immediately went into remission. My only regret is that he does not talk very much – and when he does, he sounds like everyone else.'

Broyard would like his urologist to develop a little more depth and have a bit of a sense of humour, a doctor who would appreciate both the comedy and the tragedy of his illness: 'I find an irresistible desire to make jokes. When you're lying in the hospital with a catheter and iv in your arm, you have two choices: self-pity or irony. If the doctor does not get your ironies, who else is there around?' His friends find it difficult to take this step. You don't make jokes about a serious illness. Is irony lost on cancer? In *Case Histories: Essays on Literature and Medicine*, Arko Oderwald writes that irony is one way of making fun of society's lies about a disease. 'Apart from that, in an ironic book about illness, the (self-)irony means that there are still a few laughs, which makes reading it a lot more pleasant than all those auto-biographical accounts that cannot detach themselves from immediate experience.'

More and more reports are published about nutrition and the appearance of full-blown prostate cancer, or the transformation from a pussycat into a tiger. The use of soya proteins, vitamin E and a low-fat diet supposedly protect one from prostate cancer. Precisely how that works is not yet known. As far as fats are concerned, those deriving from red meat receive a very bad press, while fish oil with its poly-unsaturated fats is not seen as harmful. The average selenium level in the Western diet is 40 micrograms, which is very little: the World Health Organization recommends between 50 and 200 micrograms a day. Ivan Wolffers, a professor of medicine, makes it clear that he feels little affinity with alternative medicine, but 'if people are really at rock bottom and for example apply endive leaves to their back with a bandage over them because they think that can restore their strength, I think: if it gives those people some peace of mind, what harm can it do?'

'Blessed is he who pees well to his dying day. No one now need suffer the agonies people once had to endure: that is a consoling thought', writes Ceronetti in *The Silence of the Body*. In his view prostate disease remains a huge drama, but at the same time he maintains that the great advance in medical science is not so much the controlling of pandemics, but the reduction in urological agony. He adds that many people live by results. 'Doctors and patients crawl from lab result to lab result, as if everything were quantifiable, but once someone has the examination result (of, say, the Prostate-Specific Antigen or PSA test) in his hands, he can never regain his innocence, he knows too much.' How true that is! How little is written about the right not to know . . .

The female prostate

Even in urological handbooks the female prostate is given very little attention. Since 1880 the organ has been known as Skene's glands. Skene was a gynaecologist and published on the subject in a medical journal. In fact, the female prostate ought to be named after the short-lived scientist Reinier de Graaf. Shortly before his death he described not only its anatomy but also its physiology. He observed that fluid was produced by women as well as men during sexual arousal and orgasm. In modern medicine it has thus far received little attention, though Professor Milan Zaviacic of the Comenius University in Bratislava, a pathologist, has made it his life's work. In 1999 he published an extensive scientific monograph on the subject.

Like the male prostate, its female counterpart produces a specific antigen (PSA), acid phosphatase, glycoproteins and fructose. The Skene glands weigh between 2.6 and 5.2 g and are located at the back of the urethra, that is, between the urethra and the vagina. Their dimensions are: on average 3.3 cm long, 1.9 cm wide and 1 cm high. There are several scores of drainage outlets from the gland tissue to the urethra, many more than in men. Zaviacic's test subjects were required to wear the same cotton panties for several days. The professor then coloured the part of the panties that had been in varying degrees of contact with the end of the urethra. Through this specific colouring it was proved that acid phosphatase, abundant quantities of which are produced in the male prostate, also flowed from the female urethra.

Various researchers have tried to discover what quantity of fluid women lose on ejaculation. The values vary from 3 to 50 millilitres on each occasion. While by no means all women can feel themselves ejaculating (estimates vary between 6 and 40%) it is probable that a form of ejaculation at orgasm is universal. Of course, researchers can capture the ejaculate for examination. If that is not possible, urine can, for example, be examined before and after an orgasm for certain substances, including PSA. The PSA content of female ejaculate averages 0.82 nanolitres per millilitre. One may speculate about the significance of the existence of the female prostate, for example for sexology, urology and gynaecology. As regards sexology, it is plausible that the Gräfenberg or G-spot, first described in the 1950s, is in fact the female prostate. For the urologist it is important to know that some 10 per cent of urethral cancers involve an adenocarcinoma, that is, prostate cancer. In addition, the female prostate quite frequently becomes inflamed, and in such cases an antibiotic is no help at all. As with men, prostatitis in women is difficult to treat: antibiotics have difficulty in penetrating the prostate.

chapter four

Testosterone and Sperm

Human testicles and those of male chimpanzees are considerably larger than those of gorillas and orang-utans, two species of ape closely related to man. Gorillas and orang-utans have modest genitalia for their large body size and ejaculate relatively meagre amounts of sperm. These animals do not require abundant quantities of sperm cells for reproduction. The male, with his silvery coat, lords it over 'his' females in the gorilla harem, and other males rarely dare take him on. This 'alpha male' does allow other males to have sex, but only with immature or pregnant females. His imposing appearance ensures that the fertile adult females remain off limits to his subordinate fellow-apes. Although orang-utans also avoid a 'sperm competition', things are slightly different with them. These solitary orange-coloured giants, which roam the forests of Borneo, have a very restrained sex life.

Comparative anatomy – the fact of man's proportionately huge testicles – indirectly illuminates the sex lives of our forefathers. Large testicles confer an advantage only where there is a sperm competition. Far back in evolution the competition to reach the ovum first was fought out between the sperm cells of various males. If two or more males mated with the same female within a few days, the one who ejaculated the largest quantity of vigorous sperm cells had the advantage in fathering descendants. Just as a car race is won by the driver with the best car, the male who mounts the female at the right moment, ejaculates most and in addition has very vigorous sperm cells, has the best chance of winning the contest. This isn't perverse: ultimately there can only be one winner, usually a type comparable with a Bugatti Veyron car, with a top speed of 400 kph and unbelievable acceleration – the envy of some male gynaecologists, so I'm told.

In *Farewell Waltz* Milan Kundera describes a cunning gynaecologist with a long nose, who treats married, childless women in a very questionable way. He gives artificial insemination using his own sperm. His professional ethics are deplorable, and he is definitely not a great lover, but genetically Kundera's doctor is the great winner. He has sired many long-nosed children for numerous happy, but deceived fathers . . . In the mid-1980s a gynaecologist in The Hague also inseminated women with his own sperm, which created a great commotion in the pages of a prestigious medical weekly. There are probably many of his offspring walking around The Hague and its environs. No trace of the inseminations, with 'fresh' instead of the usual medically checked and approved frozen sperm, could be found in the hospital records and the story was finally hushed up in a way so often convenient for doctors.

For every human being fathered in a normal way – which nowadays is no longer the case with a substantial number of people – it remains an odd idea that one has originated from one of the millions of spermatozoa that made a beeline for a single ovum. What would have happened if there had been another winner? The British cultural critic, writer and poet Aldous Huxley (1894–1963) expressed it as follows in a well-known poem ('Fifth Philosopher's Song', 1920):

> A million million spermatozoa,
> All of them alive:
> Out of their cataclysm but one poor Noah
> Dare hope to survive,
> And among that billion minus one
> Might have chanced to be
> Shakespeare, another Newton, a new
> Donne –
> But the one was Me.

It was said of the Marquis de Sade that he always carried a pillbox of sugared 'Spanish fly' with him, which he offered to unsuspecting prostitutes. Spanish fly was considered a powerful aphrodisiac, which stimulated, for example, the mucous membranes of the sex organs. This was how De Sade won his sperm wars. Research has been carried out in Britain showing that men who are aware of or suspect sexual unfaithfulness by their partners produce more powerful sperm.

Jealousy is at the same time one of the most debilitating, hate-provoking and destructive emotions. In Shakespeare's *A Winter's Tale*, Leontes, the king of Sicily, becomes totally unbalanced. Jealousy wrecks his whole life. In fact, Leontes, despite his jealous suspicions, should have taken comfort from the fact that his wife, Hermione, was pregnant. But instead every time she leaves the stage with their guest Polixenes, the king of Bohemia, Leontes becomes more distraught, more furious and more irrational. Finally he convinces himself that the child his wife is carrying is not his but the Bohemian's and obsessively examines the face of his son Mamillius for any sign of a resemblance to his Bohemian guest. Inconsolable at the doubts surrounding his paternity, Leontes orders the murder of Polixenes. He has his wife imprisoned and his son Mamillius is denied access to his mother. In prison Hermione gives birth to a daughter, whom Leontes orders to be taken into exile and abandoned. Mamillius, deprived of his mother, dies of grief, and Hermione herself falls into a death-like coma. Leontes' jealousy has destroyed not only his family but himself too: distrust and suspicion have ruined him. No one can console him or restore his confidence.

Tigers, bears and some primates do exactly the same as Leontes: they kill any young they think have been fathered by another male and so create more space among the females for their own descendants to be borne and brought up. This form of sexual selection is of course not a sperm competition; on the contrary, it is the avoidance of one.

The stickiness of sperm

Humans are descended from anthropoid primates and they in turn from mouse-like, tree-dwelling mammals. The males of some rodent species, for example the squirrel, leave behind special mating plugs. These are nothing more than a sticky, tacky secretion that prevents other males from gaining vaginal access after the first male's ejaculation. Evolution has equipped the penis of the male rodent with a special protrusion with which it can make a hole in the mating plug. Equality for all.

Male hookworms have a gland close to their sperm production centre that secretes a sticky substance. Hookworms also seal off the female's sexual orifice after successful mating. The unusual feature is that their sperm cells stay alive for a very long time, so that the female can lay the eggs fertilized by a donor even after his death. Male hookworms also use the adhesive substance to attack male rivals by sealing their genitals, so that for a while they are incapable of emitting any more sperm.

During mating the glands of Cowper in male moles swell to a tenth of their body weight, and they literally fill the female's vagina to the brim with their ejaculate. Female readers may be interested to know that in these creatures the clitoris is the same size as the penis.

The typical stickiness of human sperm is undoubtedly a remnant of the above-mentioned adhesive quality: when it dries it clings to the hair and skin. In *What is Sex?* by American biologist Lynn Margulis and journalist Dorion Sagan we are told that drones, after mating with the queen bee, forfeit their lives, leaving behind not only their genitalia but also a slimy substance. One may compare this sealing off with the frantic way in which females are guarded in some frog species. These are the ultimate sperm competition avoiders. Even if the ova have been amply fertilized by the sperm cells the males still do not let go, but cling to their partner for months on end. The writers of the above-mentioned book assume that the tough, syrupy texture of human sperm is the result of our distant mammalian origins: from mammals which had sperm that 'went hard' and acted as a kind of natural chastity belt, making access for any later would-be fertilizers difficult or even completely impossible.

Terminology

Names for sperm found on the internet include: jizz, spunk, cum, man milk, love juice, home-made yoghurt, mayo, boner brew, salt malt, cream baby juice, load, skeet, cocknog, nut-nectar, spooge and liquid sin. In a human ejaculation between 2 and 5 millilitres of sperm are emitted. Normally between 100 million and 200 million sperm cells are released on ejaculation, or between 20 and 50 million per millilitre. Sperm can be stored for years for artificial insemination, in so-called sperm banks. The sperm of animals used for breeding, like bulls and special breeds of dog, is very valuable, and millions of euros are involved in the sperm trade.

In mammals the sperm cell determines the sex of the descendant that emerges from the fertilized ovum. Techniques for sorting sperm cells by sex, so that parents can choose a boy or a girl, are being developed but are ethically controversial. This is not the case with cattle: sexed bull's sperm has been available since 2002. Despite mixed experiences in the past, use of the technique was resumed from the end of 2005. Major companies can provide sexed sperm if required. In 2005 Monsanto applied for a patent on the 'Decisive' production process, in which the sex chromosomes (X and Y) are recognized by specific colouring. Through the use of a protective thinning agent the sperm cells can survive for approximately a day in the inseminated cow.

Ejaculations

One way of explaining how an ejaculation works is by comparing it to firing a rifle. In that case too one first has to load before one can shoot, with the urethra acting as the barrel of the rifle. Ejaculation changes as one gets older: both the emission and expulsion phases last longer.

Emission stands for loading and expulsion for firing. In the emission phase the mixture of sperm cells, seminal and prostate fluid is forced into the urethra by powerful contractions of the epididymises, the sperm ducts, the seminal glands and the prostate. In the expulsion phase the prostate and the muscles beneath the urethra contract periodically and the ejaculate spurts from the penis at intervals of 0.8 seconds. Adolescents often tend to brag about how far they can 'shoot'. A certain tribe in New Guinea has turned it into a parlour game, and there are countless limericks on the subject, like the following:

> There once was a passionate pastor
> With feelings he never could master.
> His ejaculations
> Baptized congregations
> And hung from the ceiling like plaster!

In a man the amount of sperm ejaculated each time totals between 2 and 5 millilitres, after between a day and a day and a half's abstinence. According to the American urologist Metcalf the world record is half a teacup full. It is, incidentally, customary in the making of porn films for the actor who has to ejaculate to abstain for several days, so that the amount produced for the 'money shot' is as large as possible. Ask a man how many millilitres of sperm he ejaculates, and he will usually overestimate. This was certainly true of the 1970s UK band who had such hits as 'I'm Not in Love' and 'The Things We Do for Love' and called themselves 10 CC – their own estimate.

After ejaculation the sperm coagulates, becoming clotted like egg white that has been heated for a moment. After about fifteen minutes this frogspawn liquefies again.

While the sperm is being expelled the neck of the bladder is closed to prevent sperm from being forced in, as virtually always happens after a prostate operation, when the bladder can simply no longer close. The mechanism is irrevocably damaged by such a procedure, and the sperm is simply passed out with the urine.

In the elderly sensation during orgasm is greatly reduced, as happens with many other physiological processes: they run out of steam. As we get older our muscles leave us in the lurch. Much to the disappointment of patients there is nothing to be done about this. The only good piece of advice one can give is: soldier on!

How often and how soon?

'If in the first year they are together, a couple put a bean in a pot every time they make love, afterwards they will need a whole lifetime of marriage to empty the pot again if each time they make love after that first year they take a bean out of the pot,' goes a wise old Asian saying. The question of how often sexual intercourse should take place has preoccupied not only us, but also the founders of religions, philosophers and legislators.

In the Qu'ran the prophet Muhammad, who in comparison with other founders of religions shows a great deal of consideration for women, prescribes once a week. That is the woman's right, regardless of the number of wives the man has. The Jewish Talmud is less general, and distinguishes between different classes of people. The vigorous young man who is not forced to work hard is recommended to make love once a day, the ordinary workman twice a week, and scholars once a week. Professors may be given a dispensation, requiring them to have intercourse only once every two years. Martin Luther regarded twice a week as the correct quota, while the pope advises ejaculation only if there is a desire for children.

Legislators also concern themselves indirectly with frequency of intercourse. In many Western countries neither a women nor a man may be forced to have sexual intercourse within marriage. Married rape is illegal. Recent Dutch research showed that 96 per cent of couples still have intercourse once or more every two months. A problem is now arising with an increasingly frequent phenomenon, the 'double-income-no-sex syndrome'. Many couples are so wrapped up in their careers that have scarcely any time for intimacy. They regard sex as a chore to be carried out, like emptying the dishwasher.

Dr Alfred Kinsey wrote long ago that the age of the man is the most decisive factor. Kinsey was a complete number freak, and the following figures are taken from his statistics on average weekly frequency of coitus:

between 26 and 30	2.24
between 31 and 40	1.73
between 41 and 45	1.41
between 46 and 50	1.10
between 51 and 55	0.99
between 56 and 60	0.73
between 61 and 65	0.52
between 66 and 70	0.30
between 71 and 75	0.00

Kinsey's figures are pretty accurate, don't you think? Surely every reader will tend to have a quick look at his or her own age bracket, or his or her partner's.

Older men can sometimes be helped with the following rules of thumb for frequency of intercourse in relation to age:

Under 25	Twice daily
25–35	Tri-weekly
35–45	Try-weekly
45–55	Try-weakly
55–65	Try, try, try
65–76	Try anything (golf?)
75 and over	Try to remember

Many men come quickly, in their own eyes much too quickly. The modern jargon term is premature ejaculation (PE). This means that within a few seconds, or at most a minute after inserting the penis into the vagina (or another orifice) there is an ejaculation. The ejaculation may also take place during foreplay, even before insertion. Sexologists speak in such a case of *ejaculatio ante portas*. When this happens it often provokes a strong feeling of dissatisfaction and irritation, especially in one's partner.

Research in the 1940s by Kinsey and his associates showed that between 25 and 75 per cent of all adult males in the United States had an ejaculation within two minutes of penetration. That research was far less reliable than the recent multinational research led by Dutch neuro-sexologist Mark Waldinger. He is regarded as the 'inventor' of the use of the stopwatch in research into PE. The man is asked to press the button on a stopwatch at the moment of penetration so that the time it takes to reach ejaculation can be calculated exactly. In the jargon researchers speak of the Intravaginal Ejaculation Latency Time or IELT. Waldinger and his team asked 491 men, with no ailments, from Norway, Spain, Turkey, the United States and the Netherlands to participate in the stopwatch research. The average IELT turned out to be 5 minutes 40 seconds, with extremes varying in either direction from a few seconds to almost three-quarters of an hour. On the basis of the distribution curves the researchers felt able to assert that men who always climax within a minute can be regarded as 'patients', at least if they are troubled by the condition.

In any case PE is the most frequent sexual ailment in many countries. However, men seek help with it less frequently than with erectile dysfunction. Not every man sees it as a problem: for some it is a part of themselves, but with others the repeated fear of failure has a disastrous effect. People devise all kinds of tricks, varying from consuming large amounts of alcohol beforehand to thinking of rotten eggs, a herd of plodding elephants, barbed wire or blue envelopes. Another ruse is to masturbate before intercourse and hope that the second ejaculation will take slightly longer. For this purpose the man sometimes comes up with the excuse of wanting to shower before making love. Of course this makes a difference, but the disadvantage is that afterwards the arousal level may have decreased considerably. In addition, for an older man at least it takes longer to achieve a second ejaculation. None of this need be catastrophic provided the man in question ensures that his bed partner derives sufficient pleasure.

We know little about the psychological and physiological processes which cause a man to reach orgasm too quickly, though many presuppositions have been put forward. One of the first explanations was a psychoanalytical one, namely a latent hatred of women. Later psychologists decided that someone's first experiences of coitus in hasty or tense circumstances were at the root of the 'problem'. Equally, there is lack of adequate biological explanations. It is true that, for example, some rats are also 'quick off the mark'. Very probably PE is more a freak of nature. There is quite simply a gradual transition from men who come to orgasm very quickly and those who take a long time. The majority of men with PE are mentally, physically and sexually healthy and have a happy relationship with their partner. Most have no need for psychotherapy. Psychological treatment is required only if men cannot handle their PE, if the ailment has become an obsession or if their relationship with their partner has come under great pressure.

PE-sufferers can often be helped with medication, in the form of a tablet or a desensitizing cream or spray. Since the 1940s attempts have been made to make the glans and the penis less sensitive. Nowadays we use EMLA cream, usually applied to children's skins to anaesthetize them before a blood sample is taken. EMLA contains lidocaine and prilocaine, two anaesthetics. The cream must be applied at least ten minutes before intercourse, and must be wiped off in good time to prevent the partner from also becoming genitally anaesthetized. A condom can of course also be used. One annoying side-effect of the cream is that when urinating after intercourse the man may be troubled by a burning sensation at the end of the urethra. In addition the cream may cause skin rashes on the penis and the glans. Sex shops also sell anaesthetic sprays; years ago women carried similar-sized spray cans of 'intimate deodorant', which women's magazines had convinced them they needed.

It was not until the early 1970s that a medication appeared on the market that could delay ejaculation and had few side-effects. Its trade name was Anafranil and its chemical name clomipramine. Although it was easily available on prescription, little use was made of it in sexology. Only in the 1990s did treatment with pills attract widespread interest. Up to then many sexologists felt that this was simply a 'symptom-suppressant' medication, and that underlying mental problems had to be dealt with. The only snag was that in most cases there was no underlying psychological problem.

At the end of the 1980s selective serotonin re-uptake inhibitors (SSRIS) came on the market for the treatment of depression, the best-known examples being Prozac and Seroxat. In some men and women treated with certain SSRIS it was found that ejaculation or orgasm was delayed, and a number sometimes did not climax at all. In any case effect and side-effect are only words, interpretations of the result of medication. What is desirable for one person may be called a major effect. What is not desirable is quickly dismissed as a side-effect. This is what happened with SSRIS, although they are not officially indicated for PE. These types of medication should therefore be used under the supervision of a doctor.

Testicles as an aphrodisiac

Almost two thousand years ago the Latin writer Pliny recommended the eating of testicles in cases of poor sexual performance. Testes are on the menu in many countries. In Spain this delicacy is called *cojones* (with the same connotations of courage and manliness as English 'balls'). Fighting bulls from the arenas are of course the best suppliers. In the famous Florian restaurant in Barcelona they serve testicles, giving the name of the bull, its weight, a brief description, the pedigree, place and time of death and the name of the bullfighter responsible. Cojones taste of sweetbreads, but that's all that can be said: it's an illusion to think that they can be used to raise the testosterone level, since virtually all the remains of the testes will go down the drain, and the tiny amount of testosterone that is absorbed by the intestines will be immediately broken down in the liver.

Scientists

Not until the Renaissance did our knowledge of hormones and sexuality start to progress, and Paracelsus (1493–1541) became the most important scientist of the age. Theophrastus Bombastus von Hohenheim (his real name) hailed from Switzerland, and his greatest achievement was to demonstrate that many diseases could be treated and that sufferers did not always need to endure passively. He introduced mercury treatment for syphilis, the AIDS of the sixteenth century.

In the eighteenth century the English surgeon John Hunter (1728–1793) did very important and original work, being the first to observe that the testes of animals slaughtered in the autumn were smaller than those slaughtered in spring. (The reason for this has only recently been discovered. The pineal gland at the base of the brain produces more melatonin when there is more sunlight, again boosting the production of hormones in the hypophysis, which in turn prompts the testicle to produce more testosterone and sperm.) Hunter also conducted experiments with animals. After transplanting a section of a cock's testicle into a hen, he saw the hen assuming male characteristics, for example, acquiring a coxcomb. Unfortunately Hunter omitted to publish most of his findings, so that there are only sparse references to him in medical history books.

The German physiologist Berthold demonstrated in the mid-nineteenth century (1849) that when he reinserted the testicles of a castrated cockerel the creature once again developed a large comb and began behaving in a cockerel-like manner. Berthold, a professor at the University of Göttingen, wrote prolifically on every conceivable medical topic. What was his precise method? In an operation he removed the testicles of four cockerels, turning them into capons. Then he opened up the abdomen of two of the birds and implanted one testicle in each, so that that they were no longer attached to their previous nervous system. If they were to function, it would to be through the bloodstream. Berthold was incredibly lucky: antibiotics were still unknown and the capons could easily have succumbed to an inflammation of the abdominal membrane. But they survived, and the grafting of the testicles was successful. While those castrated birds in which no testicles had been replaced remained fat pacifists, the others turned back to cockerels in all respects. In his book on the male hormone Paul de Kruif puts it beautifully: 'They crowed like the proud cocks they were, they fought till the feathers flew and they chased the females enthusiastically. Their beautiful bright-red combs and dewlaps went on growing.' This was conclusive proof that the testicles fed a masculinizing substance into the blood.

Rejuvenation

Around 1900 average life expectancy increased. This was mainly due to better nutrition and hygiene. More and more people lived into middle age and beyond. Rather in the same way as in our own time, many people at the turn of the twentieth century felt the need to combat the decline that accompanies old age. It had been known since the eunuchs of Roman times that human potency is linked to the testicles, but around 1900 it was thought that vitality was also linked to them. A Viennese physiologist, Eugen Steinach, assumed that 'youth' was a product of the puberty glands, the testicles, and wrote various books on the subject.

The testicular function in older people could lead to a second youth. It wasn't really an original idea, since the celebrated physiologist Edouard Brown-Séquard (1817–1894) had already aired the same notion. He was certainly not a quack. Far from it: in his heyday the Frenchman was famed for his pioneering work in endocrinology and neurophysiology. However, the scientist could not bear the thought that he was ageing, and at the age of 70, in a desperate attempt to regain his youth, he injected himself with an extract he had made from minced rams' testicles. He immediately felt his skin tightening and firming and his mind becoming more youthful and of course recommended everyone of his age to have a jab, but was laughed out of court by his fellow scientists for having treated himself and what's more for presenting it as science.

In 1912 Steinach began his experiments with old rats. The creatures looked in poor shape, were thin and had lost their appetite for sex. Their seminal ducts were supposedly limp and empty, which made Steinbach decide to tie off their ducts and the accompanying draining blood vessels. He expected that this would result in the blood flow through the testicles increasing with a proportionate rise in testosterone production. Judging by the photos in his book, his male rats proved him right. They grew more hair, became more alert and aggressive, and their sexual interest also returned. If the treatment failed to produce the desired result, he implanted the testicles of other, young rats in the abdominal cavity or wall of the old animals and observed some degree of improvement. The rats lived twelve months longer than their usually allotted span of three years.

On 1 November the great moment came. An exhausted, emaciated Viennese workman (Anton W.) became the first human being to undergo the ligature of both seminal ducts. In the first two months after his operation there was little change, but shortly after that he improved

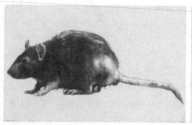 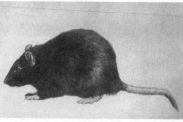

A rat before and after a rejuvenating operation.

Anton W. before
and a few months
after the tying of
his seminal ducts.

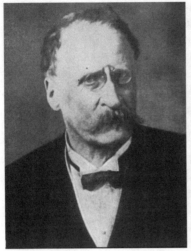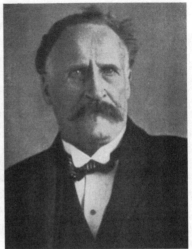

greatly. His appetite improved, he acquired more muscle bulk and was
able to resume his work. This star witness of the rejuvenating operation
walked the streets of Vienna as if reborn! Elderly gentlemen with sufficient funds soon found surgeons ready to perform the same procedure
on them. In fact, some decades previously the Italian Francesco Parona
had already reported on the injecting of veins. With a 30-year-old man
who had been impotent all his life he injected a caustic substance into
a kind of varicose vein on the penis. By the fifth day after the operation
the patient had had sex five times!

Steinach was regarded as a charlatan by many of his colleagues,
but in the meantime he had acquired Sigmund Freud as a patient. He
himself was well aware of the limitations of his experiments, since the
research field of ageing, impotence and possible hormonal effects was
far too complex for one humble researcher. Others would continue his
work.

In the same period Serge Voronoff began causing a stir with testicle extracts. After various travels in Africa, this eccentric, flamboyant
Russian became head of the then renowned experimental laboratory
at the Collège de France. While working as a surgeon in Algiers he had
become interested in the welfare of castrated boys, whom he found
both mentally and physically retarded. Young patients with tuberculosis of their sex organs were mostly castrated at the time, and as a result,
so Voronoff believed, after some years suffered loss of memory and
poor concentration. In addition, he had never known a eunuch to live
beyond 60. For this reason he formulated the hypothesis that the loss
of the testicles accelerated the occurrence of signs of ageing. He was
firmly convinced that old testicles needed support, but unfortunately

the Steinach operation had ultimately produced too few satisfied patients. What's more, Voronoff had shown irrefutably by experiment that transplanting young testicles under the skin of the abdomen did not help either. Without an adequate blood supply the testicles soon failed. Vascular surgery was still in its infancy: nowadays blood vessels can if necessary be sewn together with the aid of a microscrope.

Voronoff therefore decided on a different approach from his Viennese colleague. He took testicular tissue, cut it into thin slices and placed it in the fleshy casing of the existing testicle, after first scratching that casing with his scalpel, in the hope that this stimulus would cause new blood vessels to form, thus providing nutrition for the transplant. However, the most spectacular thing about his method was the donor. Whereas Steinach's followers used the undescended testicles of young men, Voronoff favoured ape testicles.

In June 1920 he performed his first transplant, followed within a few years by three hundred others all over the world. By 1927 the figure had risen to over a thousand! Whether the transplant had taken could only be confirmed by microscopic examination. But who would sacrifice his feeling of being 'reborn' for the sake of science? In 1923 the Russian had personally performed over forty operations, half of them on patients under the age of 60. Of course, these were not just any patients: they included professors, architects, writers and industrialists. For years they wrote letters about their young appearance and sexual potency! Predictably, Voronoff also transplanted testicles into homosexuals with the aim of 'curing' them. Like Steinach, Voronoff was scarcely taken seriously by official medicine, but this miracle-worker nevertheless became a worldwide celebrity among randy old men.

A contemporary Russian writer incorporated the theme of rejuvenation and testicle transplantation into his work, but turning the process on its head, he imagined a transplant from man to animal. Mikhail Bulgakov (1890–1940) studied medicine and worked for a short time as a village doctor. His only literary work published in full in the former Soviet Union during his lifetime is a collection of satirical stories, *Heart of a Dog*. In one of them a professor, who has more or less managed to escape the dictatorship of the proletariat, is working on rejuvenation experiments. He implants the testicles and pineal gland of a recently deceased, disreputable musician into a dog. The dog gradually turns into a loud, foul-mouthed human being. What's more, he becomes close friends with the fanatical chairman of the residents' committee, who is determined to destroy the professor and his prosperity. Under the influence of the fanatical chairman the dog becomes increasingly disobedient to its creator. The professor realizes his error and returns the dog to its original state. In this way he intends to rescue

Chair for testicle
diathermia
procedure.

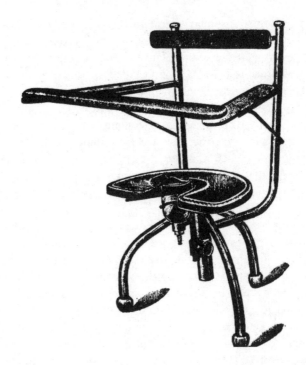

mankind from monsters like the doggish proletarian with his Marxist-Leninist pronouncements. The story is full of both science fiction and satire, and the indirect critique of Bolshevism is quite obvious.

The French doctor Denis Courtade believed, like many contemporaries, that application of all kinds of electricity – faradic or galvanic – to different parts of the body – head, sacrum, lumbar vertebrae – could cure impotence. In cases of impotence through inflammation of the prostate an internal rectal electrode was inserted. The next step was application of diathermia to the testicles. By raising the temperature of the testes slightly it was hoped to boost the secretion of testosterone, and a special chair had been designed for the purpose. A hole at the front of a glass allowed the scrotum to be suspended in a saline solution, after which electrical stimulation could begin. The treatment was given three or four times a week for a month. That was enough: even then it was known that a long-term rise in temperature could lead to a reduction in sperm production.

Developments in America were almost identical to those in Europe. There too the tying off of the arteries of the scrotum was the first surgical treatment for impotence. The surgeon James Duncan published on the subject in March 1895. A 66-year-old impotent widower, who had found Spanish fly ineffective, was the first victim. The operation took place under local anaesthetic (cocaine). Duncan's fellow surgeon

Wooten performed a similar operation in 1902 and wrote a verbose article about it. In 1908 the urologist Professor Lydston stated that the positive results were due to the relative impedence of drainage and the resulting enlarged testicles: 'The larger the testicles are after the operation, the more impressed the patient is. He believes that the operation has been successful and his self-confidence returns. The positive results turn out to be mostly lasting, even after complications have developed in the long term', wrote the professor from Illinois. Despite his optimistic pronouncements, however, the operation was soon forgotten. The fact was that the long-term outcomes were dire. Nevertheless Lowsley continued the treatment until 1953, operating on thousands of men.

A certain Professor Lespinasse, though, managed to transplant testicular tissue from recently deceased men into the abdominal muscles of living impotent men. Whenever anyone had committed suicide or been executed, Lespinasse was on the scene in a flash to remove the testicles. Meanwhile the impotent recipient of the donor tissue was prepared for operation by his assistants. Unfortunately the transplant was invariably rejected. Up to now there have been very few successful attempts to transplant a testicle stalk and all. In every case the transplantation involved monozygotic twins, one of whom had no testicles and the other two.

A young prison doctor in San Quentin named Leo Stanley had an easier time in 1918. He implanted the testes of executed inmates into prisoners in various age groups to see if in this way he could effectively treat acne and asthma. His test subjects, though, received no remission of sentence.

The quest

American doctors performed many other odd experiments. The book *The Male Hormone* tells the story of Professor Fred Koch and his student Lemuel McGee, both employed at the University of Chicago. They cheerfully mashed, extracted, fractionized and distilled thousands of kilograms of bulls' testicles, in search of the pure male sex hormone. From 40 kg of testicles they obtained 20 mg of impure but active substance. The effort was disproportionate: 40 kg for a few paltry milograms, and a narrowly failed attempt to win the Nobel Prize.

In 1929 it was the turn of human beings: a 26-year-old man with scarcely any pubic hair, no moustache or beard and with a high-pitched voice was treated with the substance for 53 days. And lo and behold, he was transformed into a real man! He also developed a normal sexual appetite with orgasm and ejaculation. The ultimate proof of the importance of the male sex hormone! However, disillusion followed, since it would never be possible to obtain enough bulls' testicles for commercial use. Apart from which the processing of the testicles cost a fortune.

The dynamic German chemist Adolf Butenlandt took a different tack: he worked for the Schering chemical group and collected thousands of litres of urine, produced by policemen – over 25,000 litres in all. He knew that this must contain the active substance. Eventually he obtained a few crystals consisting mainly of androsterone, a decomposition product of testosterone.

On 27 May 1935 the chemist Ernst Laqueur succeeded in determining the exact structural formula of the sex hormone. He led an excellent research team at the Organon company, and was also a professor of pharmacology at Amsterdam University. He called the hormone testosterone, and the title of his famous article was 'On crystalline male hormone from testicles'. Laqueur too had unfortunately

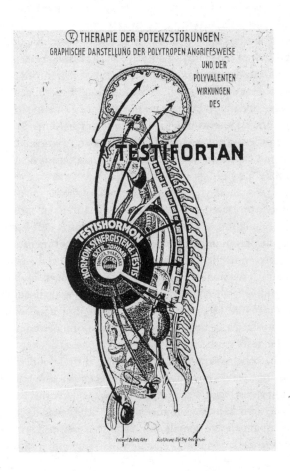

Testifortan,
an impotence
remedy.

required kilograms of bulls' testicles. At that point the miracle happened that so many scientists had been hoping for: it was found that cholesterol could be converted synthetically into testosterone. In no time there were several manufacturers. The discovery was the achievement of the chemist Leopold Ružička, who worked for the Swiss firm of Ciba. Cod liver oil and sheep's fat, both rich in cholesterol, became the main raw materials. Butenlandt and Ružička were awarded the Nobel Prize in 1939, but Laqueur's work went unrecognized.

How is testosterone viewed today, and what do scientists know about it? Testosterone is a compound of testis and steroid. Its systematic name is 17beta-hydroxy-4-androsten-3-on. The blood contains a large store of testosterone, a hundred times more than is found in those places where it should be active. This reserve in the blood is attached to transport proteins, which release it only when there is a demand.

A very large number of animal species produce testosterone, but in all females the amount of testosterone is considerably lower than in males. In the womb testosterone ensures that the embryo develops into a boy and during puberty it is responsible for the appearance of secondary male sexual characteristics (including the breaking of the voice, and the growth of the penis, scrotum, pubic hair and skeletal muscles). After puberty testosterone also maintains the male reproductive apparatus, the male body shape and the production of sperm cells. Because it strengthens the muscular system, it is banned from sport. The principal male hormone also plays a part in men's balding. In both men and women it ensures a healthy libido and also promotes the growth of female pubic hair. In men testosterone is produced in the adrenal glands and by the Leydig cells in the testicles, between 5 and 7 mg per day in all. In women the production is a tenth of that in men. In women testosterone is produced in the ovaries, in the adrenal glands and fatty tissue. The regulation of testosterone is very complex. It begins in the hypothalamus. From puberty onwards, besides its other functions, the hypothalamus transmits increasing numbers of special signals to the hypophysis. These signals (GnRH, gonadotrophine-stimulating hormone) prompt the hypophysis in turn to pass on special signals to the testes by means of FSH – follicle-stimulating hormone – and LH – luteinizing hormone. When the concentrations of FSH and LH are high enough, the testes produce more testosterone. The hypothalamus measures the concentrations of testosterone in the blood; when these exceed a certain level, the hypothalamus transmits a different signal to the hypophysis, so that the production of testosterone is inhibited. Testosterone is broken down in the liver. In both the Leydig and Sertoli cells small quantities of female hormone (oestrogens) are produced from testosterone.

The feedback mechanisms.

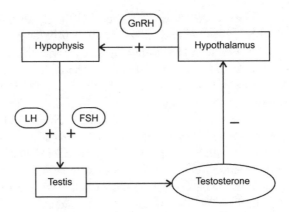

A serious depletion of testosterone is caused, for example, by certain diseases of the hypothalamus and abnormalities in the testicles, for instance in men with Klinefelter's syndrome, and certain kidney diseases. Obese men with diabetes also often have too low a testosterone level (see the following section). If the hormone level is completely normal, there is no point in administering additional testosterone, which only creates additional risks of side-effects such as liver abnormalities and the activation of latent prostate cancer.

Testicular pension?

Men of sixty are often determined to prove their masculinity, basically because they have very little left. The pious King David in the Bible was no exception, when from his roof terrace he saw Bathsheba, the wife of Uriah, one of his bravest and most loyal commanders, taking a bath (II Samuel 11:2). In a wave of passion he had her summoned and seduced her. However, when Bathsheba, who was quite flattered by the king's attentions, became pregnant, David lost no time in recalling her husband from the battlefield, where he had been for months, in order to pass off the child as his. Uriah, as a dutiful soldier, refused to return. The king devised a ruse. He had a message delivered to the general with the request that Captain Uriah be sent to the palace in Jerusalem. Uriah came and was most warmly received. The king inquired with interest about the course of events at the front, and also inquired about the general's state of health. Uriah must have found this very odd, since it was most unusual to recall a junior officer from the front in order to report to the king. A monarch discussed important military matters with his most senior commanders.

David thanked Uriah fulsomely, gave him a splendid gift and sent him back home, close to the palace. The intention was clear: David wanted the sexually deprived Uriah to take his Bathsheba in a passionate embrace, and later discover that he had fathered an eight-month or seven-month child with her. Imagine David's dismay when he learned that Uriah had not gone home, but had lain down to sleep among the palace staff at the entrance to the palace. David immediately summoned Uriah again and asked him why he hadn't simply gone home to bed. His reply was typical of an upright professional soldier:

'Your Majesty,' said Uriah, 'my troops and even my general are camped in the field, and are sleeping on the ground, or at best in a tent. It would have been unbecoming if I were to sleep with my wife.'

It was not only the decency of the simple captain that thwarted the king's evil plan. We know that at this period sexual abstinence during military campaigns was regarded as a religious duty. The king dreamt up a new ruse. He persuaded Uriah to stay a day longer in Jerusalem and invited him to dinner. He managed to get Uriah drunk, but it was no good. Even in his cups, the captain stuck to his principles and refused to go home. Again he lay down to sleep among the palace servants. Because of his decency he had unwittingly signed his own death warrant.

The king had no choice but to manoeuvre the dutiful captain into such a position on the battlefield that his death in combat was inevitable. A dastardly trick! But God punished him for it, immediately. After his crime the king could find no rest. At the age of seventy he was a broken man, and rumour circulated throughout Israel that the king was completely finished. There was even talk of deposing him. Naturally his courtiers were alarmed: proof of his virility was needed, so that the monarchy could be saved! For this purpose they fetched a very beautiful virgin, called Abisag, from Sunem, about 13 km south of Nazareth. She became his personal nurse, companion and carer. At night she slept with him and with her warm young body drove the cold out of David's stiff old frame.

Humiliatingly, however, the king could not manage to have intercourse with her. The rumour about his impotence spread throughout Israel; Bathsheba profited from his weakness and forced David to appoint her second son Solomon as his successor. And Solomon grew in power and strength and according to tradition had a thousand wives . . .

Why this wonderful biblical story? Well, in the view of modern scientists the king, with his declining sexual powers, was suffering from what today is called the male climacteric, or andropause. Strictly speaking there is no such thing as a climacteric in the ageing man. With men there is no sudden shutdown of the sex glands as is the case with women. The same applies to fertility, which is of course less great than when they were young, but even so . . . Anthony Quinn, Pablo Picasso,

Charlie Chaplin, Yves Montand and Marlon Brando are well-known examples of men who became fathers late in life.

In men there is no abrupt cessation of testosterone production, more a gradual reduction. At the age of 75 it is only half of what it was at the age of 30. That reduction may be accompanied by loss of libido, forgetfulness, sleep disturbance, depression, loss of muscle mass and strength, loss of elasticity in the skin, osteoporosis and increased risk of cardiovascular disease. Experts estimate that there is a testosterone deficiency in between 20 and 30 per cent of men between thirty and eighty. As regards the other hormones: the concentration of DHEA (dehydropiandrosterone), which is produced in the adrenal gland, is only one-third of that in 25-year-olds. Oestrogen serum levels remain constant because of an increase in body fat; one result of that often seen in ageing men is the formation of breasts. The secretion of melatonin from the pineal gland is also reduced in older men.

Testosterone supplements?

For decades the reduction of sex hormones in post-menopausal women has been the subject of study and for decades women presenting with associated problems have been treated with female hormones. Nowadays a deficiency of active androgens like testosterone in men is known not as andropause but as PADAM, or Partial Androgen Deficiency in the Ageing Male. Every ten years those in the field dream up a new acronym. The term 'penopause' is, however, no longer current.

In contrast to the position with women, treatment of the ageing man with a deficiency of androgens is still in its infancy. Administering testosterone to ageing men may have a favourable effect on the previously mentioned symptoms. But what men should be treated? Up to now there has been no research on which to base an adequate answer to this question. The administering of testosterone to ageing men with 'normal' testosterone levels in their blood serum but with a typical pattern of symptoms is currently the subject of debate, but unfortunately the research that has been carried out has been with 'healthy' older men and there have been no double-blind placebo-controlled studies. In the latter the effects of a possible drug are compared with those of a placebo, where neither the researcher nor the test subject knows which drug is being administered or taken.

As indicated by the term PADAM, older men suffer only from a partial deficiency, which fact needs supplementing only to the normal level. Until recently that could be done only with capsules or injections. The use of skin patches is also possible, but the best way appears to be the daily application of a gel to the chest and shoulders. Two makes are available commercially, one smelling of perfume, the other of pure alcohol – take your pick. Finally, testosterone can also be administered via a bio-adhesive tablet on the gum above the upper incisor teeth.

Testosterone and drug-taking in sport

Testosterone was one of the first performance-enhancing drugs to be used in sport. In combination with strength training it is a powerful muscle strengthener, an anabolic. When scientists succeeded in manufacturing the hormone synthetically it fairly soon became all the rage among sportsmen. But not only sportsmen: Adolf Hitler and other top Nazi leaders became users. Servicemen were given doses to increase their belligerence and aggression. The mafioso Al Capone's devotion to the drug accounted for his hoarse voice.

American research blew the whistle: testosterone and the derived anabolic steroids turned out to have too many side-effects. But athletes had realized that these 'sweets' helped enhance their performance, and the ban on use was flouted. During the world weightlifting championships of 1954 the coach of the losing team discovered this in an odd way. Several Russian weightlifters could no longer urinate normally, but had to insert a catheter to empty their bladders. After the victory, a tipsy Russian explained: as a result of daily injections of testosterone the prostate had swollen so much that the urethra was squeezed shut. There were no drug checks in those days, and meanwhile certain pharmaceutical companies steadily improved synthetic testosterone: injections became unnecessary and were replaced by pills, which proved to have less effect on the prostate. Bodybuilders, weightlifters, swimmers and racing cyclists flocked to take the wonder pills. The potential benefits of testosterone and its derivatives have probably been nowhere as thoroughly researched as in the former German Democratic Republic before the fall of the Iron Curtain. Whole series of theses appeared on the subject at Marxist universities.

On average the testicles produce between 5 and 7 mg of testosterone per day. If over and above that one administers testosterone in high doses, for example an extra 25 mg, the blood testosterone level scarcely changes, since the hormone is rapidly broken down in the liver. In order to achieve a really positive effect substances were developed that acted in the same way as testosterone, but were not broken down so quickly in the liver. These molecules, which were chemically closely related to testosterone, were called anabolic steroids. Examples include methandrostenolon, oxandrolon, danazol and tanazol.

Abuse has been and remains widespread. Many users are young, insecure men, who use anabolic steroids, in combination with physical workouts, to train not only their body but their mind. Unfortunately that is not the end of the story. Anabolic steroids turn the body's hormone economy upside down: cartilage growth increases, causing, for example, the Adam's apple to widen and the vocal cords to lengthen, so that the voice becomes first hoarser and subsequently lower. Body hair increases and women develop beards and moustaches, while in both men and women the hair on the scalp thins. The skin becomes thicker and greasier as a result of the increased number of sebaceous glands, so that anabolic steroid users suffer more from acne. In women the breasts tend to sag and the clitoris increases in size – the latter effect is irreversible and the organ, which is normally mostly hidden, will become more prominent. Pregnancy while using anabolic steroids is a risky business: a female foetus has a good chance of being born with masculine features. Fortunately, in the great majority of cases women using anabolic steroids will not succeed in becoming pregnant.

Men disrupt their hormone economy to such an extent that their own testosterone production decreases or completely stops. This is because the hypothalamus, the centre in the brain that regulates and adjusts testosterone production, receives the signal that more than enough testosterone is circulating in the body. The problem is that anabolic steroids differ from testosterone in that they cannot regulate sperm production, with the result that men become infertile. All men produce a small amount of female hormone, though in a healthy body that is only a tiny fraction compared with testosterone, but if an individual's own testosterone production stops, the female hormones increase in importance, resulting in shrinking testicles and breastformation.

Male hormonal contraception

The concentration of testosterone is many times greater in the testes than in serum. Unlike in other androgen-dependent organs, such as the prostate and seminal glands, a multiple of the serum concentration in the testes is also necessary for normal functioning (spermatogenesis). Grateful use is made of this phenomenon in research into a male contraceptive. If testosterone is administered to a man the secretion of, for example, luteinizing hormone (LH) by the hypophysis will be greatly inhibited. Testosterone secretion by the Leydig cells is brought virtually to a halt. A dose of 200 mg of testosterone per week, injected into the lumbar muscle, results in a doubling of testosterone levels. Partly through the inhibition in the Leydig cells and the accompanying fall of the testosterone level in the testes, sperm cell production virtually ceases.

As a young man the Groningen-based researcher Pek van Andel devised a method of measuring sperm production in rats: he severed the seminal ducts as far downstream as possible and implanted them directly into the bladder. In this way it was possible to monitor exactly how many sperm cells a rat produced daily, a process that Pek described in his first publication. He was later to win the alternative Nobel Prize for his idea of using an MRI scanner in which couples could have intercourse as a research tool.

In the spring of 2006 *The Lancet*, one of the world's most authoritative medical journals, surveyed the state of research. It had been shown that the male version of hormonal contraception was safe and reversible. The study concerned had involved over 1,500 men. The researchers found that the average time required for sperm to recover to a level of 20 million spermatozoa per millilitre (the level at which one speaks of a 'normal' sperm count), was between three and four months. Older men, men of Asian origin, men with a high sperm level at the start of the study and men who had used hormonal contraception for only a short time, recovered quickest. The figures: 67 per cent recovered within six months, 90 per cent within twelve months, 96 per cent within sixteen months and 100 per cent were back to their original level after two years. According to the authors of the article in this leading publication their study had proved that the previously demonstrated efficacy of hormonal contraception was accompanied by a high degree of sperm recovery. New research is underway in which an androgen like testosterone is combined with a progestagen.

Testosterone and women

Testosterone production in women, as in men, is variable in several respects. Just after birth girls produce relatively large amounts of testosterone. Production declines throughout childhood and increases again with the onset of puberty. Testosterone levels peak around the age of 30, after which there is a steady decline. Women of around forty produce only half the amount of testosterone produced by those in their twenties. Testosterone production also fluctuates with the menstrual cycle: around ovulation the concentration is obviously highest, which is also when women feel most like having sex. It has also been shown that women have small day-to-day fluctuations: testosterone concentration in the blood is highest at about ten in the morning, and falls again through the day.

In his book *De Mietjesmaatschappij* (The Sissy Society, 2000), science journalist Marcel Roele writes that housewives produce on average less male hormone than career women. If one compares different kinds of working woman, women who are employed as PAs, nurses or primary schoolteachers have less testosterone than women doctors, lawyers or managers. The more testosterone, the greater the competitive urge? Who can say? In *De Pikorde* (The Pecking Order, 2006) Marleen Finoulst and Dirk Vanderschueren report that years ago a British gynaecologist had prescribed testosterone to five of the then 118 female MPs, in the hope that this would help them compete better with their male colleagues on committees and in parliamentary debates. The female politicians gave this idea short shrift and protested that they had no need of testosterone!

In the menopause, when activity in the ovaries slowly fades, the production of testosterone also declines. Yet after the change women often have to deal with unwanted hair growth, for example on the upper lip and around the chin, while the hair on their head tends to thin. That is mainly because the liver produces less transport proteins, so releasing more free testosterone. The free form is the 'active' one, so that despite the falling hormone production the relative quantity of active testosterone in creases. This is why unwanted masculinizing features occur.

In the United States menopausal women are regularly prescribed testosterone. Over 30 per cent of older American women take hormone pills and in half of these cases the pills contain testosterone. In many other countries that is still highly unusual. A drop in normal testosterone levels may, as has been said, be the result of the menopause, but also, for instance, of the removal of both ovaries and chemotherapy. In such cases women may suffer acute listlessness, a reduction in muscle power, loss of pubic hair, loss of sexual appetite and may find it difficult or impossible to achieve orgasm. Giving testosterone supplements only makes sense if there really is a deficiency. Similarly, menopausal problems like vaginal dryness and hot flushes are not treated with testosterone; oestrogens are used for this purpose. The same phenomenon is found in those taking the contraceptive pill: taking extra female hormones leads to a decrease in testosterone production.

chapter five

Castration

Today, when most people hear the word 'eunuch', their first associations are with weakness, sexual impotence, inadequacy as a man, etc. That has definitely not been the case throughout history. To judge by the alarmed reaction to the very word, you'd never think that castration was once a popular practice. But it was: for centuries men had themselves voluntarily castrated, for a whole variety of motives. The eunuch, originally imported as a slave, gradually transcended his image of bondage. Eunuchs were considered to be very loyal: after all, they had had no other family than their master, they had been abducted from parents and homeland and could not father any descendants of their own. In general eunuchs proved extremely faithful and devoted, but there were many potential rewards for their servitude. Eunuchs worked as opera singers, choristers, generals, theologians, philosophers, chamberlains, prophets, harem guards, tutors to imperial children, tax inspectors – the list is endless. In this way they served imperial families, the aristocracy and religious institutions and were certainly neither puny nor pathetic.

Archaeologists believe that the castration of animals began in around 4500–4000 BC. Animal husbandry, which had begun with sheep, pigs and goats, was extended to cattle. Bulls were not only an important source of meat, but also provided muscle power for pulling ploughs and carts. The only problem was that bulls could not be kept together. The magic solution turned out to be castration, and the ox was born. Increased manageability was a motive for the castration of many domesticated animals. Castration of tomcats prevented them from spraying urine all over the house and also had a calming effect on their behaviour.

No so long ago, in order to help dogs deal better with the psychological effects of their castration, an American company (CTI Corporation, Bruckner, Missouri), brought out a product called Neuticles: testes prosthetics for dogs. The manufacturer stressed that with this product a dog would look just the same after the operation as before, while the animal would feel the same and wouldn't really know that it had been castrated. Bumper stickers carrying the slogan 'I love Neuticles' were printed for the cars of proud dog-owners! In the case of a number of domesticated species of animal special names were devised for castrated individuals: a stallion or a male donkey became a gelding, a boar (male pig) a barrow, a ram a wether and a cock a capon. As has been said, primitive man soon realized that castration of his animals could prove beneficial. It made animals easier to fatten and easier to handle. Castrated animals usually abandoned their normal behaviour: geldings proved more suitable for riding and driving, capon meat was more plentiful and juicier, and schnitzels made from barrows were tastier. Over the centuries oxen were used less and less as draught animals, but because oxen store more fat in their muscle tissue, castration remained in vogue, since once slaughtered they provided better beef.

Nowadays male piglets are castrated when they are two weeks old. Before then the piglets are too young to survive the procedure, and if one waits too long, only a vet can carry out the castration. The set of forceps used for the castration is called an *emasculator*. With calves and lambs the seminal cords may be severed using a so-called *burdizzo* up to the age of two months – all without anaesthetic.

The term castration is probably derived from the Latin *castor*, beaver, since the latter is said to bite off its own testicles when in danger. It was as if beavers were surrendering their *castoreum*, and so saving their lives. By the middle of the nineteenth century the beaver had been all but wiped out in Europe because of the castoreum secreted by their anal glands, which commanded extraordinarily high prices. It was used to treat not only impotence, but toothache and heart problems, and it was also smeared on beehives to increase the honey yield.

Gary Taylor has written an amusing history of castration (*Castration: An Abbreviated History of Western Manhood*), based on religion, biology, anthropology, etc. One can forgive Taylor for becoming slightly ponderous when he tries to situate castration theoretically, but having read his book, one thinks: all things considered, the balls on the Christmas tree are the ultimate symbol of the international annexation of pagan ideas by Christians.

The human fear of castration is very deep-seated, more so than most people think. In Greek mythology it is referred to a number of times, for example in the story of Uranus and Melampus. The noble parts of Uranus, having been thrown into the sea, brought forth Venus, and

Melampus was later involved in curing a prince (Iphiclus) who suffered from impotence and was unable to father children – an affliction also caused by castration anxiety.

The myth of Melampus and Iphiclus

Melampus means 'black-foot'. His feet were black because although his mother had placed him in the shade shortly after his birth, she had carelessly left his feet exposed to the sunlight. From an early age Melampus was fond of all animals. In front of his father's house was a large oak and a hollow at its base was home to two snakes. The creatures were quite harmless and Melampus was fascinated by them, especially when he noticed that there were young on the way. These had no sooner been born than his father's servant beat the two adult snakes to death. The grief-stricken Melampus burned the dead snakes and carefully reared their orphaned brood. One day, when they were fully grown, the snakes slid to his bedside and licked his ears with their tongues. The startled Melampus sat bolt upright . . . and immediately could hear what birds flying overhead were saying to each other. From then on he could foretell the future, since the birds told him everything that was about to happen. On the banks of the River Alpheus he met the god Apollo and became an accomplished seer.

As luck would have it, Melampus' brother Bias had set his sights on the delectable Pero, but her father refused to give her in marriage to anyone but the man who could bring him Phulakos' herd of cattle. The problem was that the herd was guarded by a dog too fierce to be approached by man or beast. At his wit's end, Bias asked his omniscient brother for help. Melampus agreed to try. He foresaw that he would be caught in the act and put in prison, but would return with the herd.

Things turned out just as he had predicted, and a married couple were appointed as his jailers. The husband treated him with great kindness, while the wife behaved viciously towards the shackled prisoner. Then something very odd happened! Up in the wooden roof Melampus heard woodworm talking to each other. From their conversation he gathered that they had very nearly eaten their way through the main roof beam. Melampus hurriedly called his guards, claiming that he felt ill and preferred not to remain in the low-ceilinged room. They lifted his bed, with the husband at the head and the wife at the foot. As they were carrying him outside the woman was struck a fatal blow by the falling beam.

Of course the husband reported the incident to Phulakos, the owner of the herd. Phulakos went to see the prisoner with his son Iphiclus and asked Melampus who he really was. When Melampus replied that he was a seer, he was immediately released from his shackles and invited to the royal citadel. The king asked Melampus to cure his son, who was unable to sire children. Melampus agreed, on condition that if he proved successful he would be rewarded with the herd.

The seer then sacrificed a bull, cut the meat into small pieces and invited all the birds except for the reclusive vulture to come and eat. They all flocked to the feast and Melampus asked each one about the secret cure for Iphiclus' ailment. The birds did not know, but when they noticed the vulture was not yet in their midst, they went and fetched him. The old vulture arrived and told his story:

> One day Phulakos was with the herd, castrating new-born bull-calves with a knife. Iphiclus, then still a child, was with him and had been misbehaving, causing his father to fly into a rage and push the knife against his son's genitalia. To frighten the boy still further he had thrown the knife up into a tree. It had lodged in the tree and the bark had grown over it. This gave Iphiclus such a terrible shock that ever since he had been impotent and unable to sire children.

The old vulture said that the king's son could be cured; the knife must be recovered from beneath the bark of the oak, rust must be scraped off it and Iphiclus must drink a glass of wine containing the rust scrapings for a period of ten days.

Melampus found the knife and the magic potion proved effective. Nine months later Iphiclus' son was born. He was named Podarkes, 'swift-foot', because his father had excelled as a sportsman since childhood. The joyful Melampus took the herd and Bias to meet the bride his brother had longed for so passionately . . .

Freud and castration anxiety

The story of Oedipus, who unwittingly killed his father and equally unwittingly married his mother, is widely known. This led Sigmund Freud to use Oedipus' name for a discovery he made in his consulting room concerning the human subconscious. Freud sees the Oedipal phase as commencing when the child is between three and five. He also calls this the phallic phase, a time in which the external sex organs are central to the child's mental map. At the same time this phase sees the emergence of the superego, the conscience, beginning with the internalizing of parental authority – for boys mainly the father's – and is hence also the point at which guilt feelings may arise.

Two central concepts in Freud's theory are castration anxiety in boys and girls and penis envy in girls. Castration anxiety leads the boy to defer to his father, while penis envy causes the girl to focus on her father. After a period in which children's principal attachment is to the mother, the father figure comes more into the picture. In boys this results in an ambivalent feeling towards the father: rivalry and anxiety on the one hand, admiration and protectiveness on the other. The boy would love to give his mother a baby, and resolves this ambivalence by identifying with his father and emulating him, which is how he becomes a man. For a girl it means an intense focus on the father; she would like a penis too and would love to have his baby or give her mother a baby. The young girl experiences these as the same thing. She becomes ambivalent towards the mother: she distances herself somewhat, but is also frightened of losing her mother. The girl resolves this ambiguity by identifying with the mother and emulating her. In Freud's view this is how the girl becomes a woman.

Castration in China

An ancient Chinese term for eunuch was *huan kuan*: a castrated man employed in the palace. In imperial China there was widespread castration of young boys. The local and provincial nobility imitated the emperor and also kept eunuchs. Many parents sent their sons to the courts in the hope of later benefits. This resulted in the creation of a very special occupation: that of castrator. He removed the whole penis and scrotum, after which the boy's urine was channelled through a straw. Following the operation, performed without anaesthetic (!), some boys became incontinent. The castrator kept the penis and testicles, which the eunuch could later redeem at a high price; many eunuchs wished to be buried 'whole'.

In the late Ming and Qing periods these castrati were notorious for their corruption. Since eunuchs were the only men allowed in the emperor's private quarters, a young emperor would frequently develop a strong bond of trust with them. In practice they were closely involved with the upbringing of the children at the imperial court. The eunuchs reached the apogee of their power during the Ming dynasty, when they controlled virtually all administrative posts. They not only promulgated laws, but also chose the concubines and even the wife of the emperor. Palace eunuchs became so rich that they had luxurious palaces built in their native regions. Most of them were from the Beijing area or the Hebei peninsula and a few came from Shandong province or Mongolia.

The conflict between the corrupt eunuch and the virtuous Confucian official who resists his tyranny became a commonplace in

Chinese historiography. In his *History of Government* Samuel Finer observes perceptively that the reality was often less black and white. There were very competent eunuchs, who proved valuable advisors to their emperor, while the resistance of the 'virtuous' official was not infrequently the blind resistance of a member of a privileged caste, opposed to all radical change, regardless of whether it was harmful or salutary for the country. But then, in China history books were generally written by officials.

The Ottoman Empire

Like the Chinese emperor the Ottoman sultans kept eunuchs, though these were imported slaves. Since Sharia law forbade mutilation of the human body, they were castrated by non-Muslim traders outside Islamic territory. Recent research by M. W. Aucoin and R. J. Wasserzug has shown that in early-medieval Islamic territory eunuchs were active heterosexually and homosexually, in the latter case in both passive and active roles.

At the end of the sixteenth century the Turks chose eunuchs principally from among white slaves of Slav, German or Hungarian origin. Later they were supplied mainly by the monastery of Abou Gerbè in Upper Egypt, where Coptic priests castrated dark-skinned Nubian or Abyssinian boys, usually at the age of eight. The operation was a radical one, in which the whole scrotum, the testicles and the penis were removed, and the death rate was high. In his lavishly illustrated book *From Seduction to Mutilation*, my fellow urologist Johan Mattelaer reveals how lucrative the trade in eunuchs was: traders negotiated with African tribal chiefs, who regarded their boys as nothing but merchandise. These young slaves were transported via the Nile or the Red Sea, and castration was usually carried out at a staging post, never by Muslims, as was said, but usually by Jews or Christians. The surgery was performed without any precautionary measures. Hot desert sand was the only remedy in the case of bleeding. This valuable merchandise virtually never reached the slave markets, but was sold en route and set to work in the Topkapi palace in Constantinople. There was a distinction between black and white: dark-skinned eunuchs had more successful careers. The young white boys of Christian origin carried out mainly domestic tasks and were not allowed to guard the harems, a task reserved for black eunuchs, preferably with ugly, scarred faces, so that any trace of sexual interest from the residents of the harem would be nipped in the bud. They had to check who entered, accompany the women on their rare outings, and act as intermediaries in contacts with the outside world. The head of the black eunuchs was an important man, the right hand and confidant of the sultan-mother, and in addition he was allowed to approach the sultan without an intermediary, a privilege granted to only a few. He had to supply new concubines for the harem, pronounced the death sentence and officiated personally at executions.

The political power of the eunuchs was greatest at the end of the sixteenth century, after which their influence declined, and after the political reforms at the end of the nineteenth century their duties were limited to receiving ladies wishing to visit the harem and escorting their mistresses on their visits to the bazaar. In 1909 the harem was closed and the sultan was compelled to release his eunuchs.

India

In the ancient Hindu tradition patients with metastasized prostate cancer were treated by the same method used by many of today's urologists, namely chemical castration. Nowadays this is done with expensive pills or depot injections, while in the past a cheap, vegetarian diet was used. This was very low in cholesterol, by far the most important raw material used by our bodies for the production of testosterone. Once castrated the patient found it easier to observe complete sexual abstinence, freeing more energy for spiritual ends. Think of the time we would save if we were castrated. In fact research has confirmed that a low-fat diet causes the testosterone level in the blood to drop by approximately 10 per cent, though certainly not to what urologists call 'castration level'.

India has an estimated million-plus eunuchs. Many have been castrated before puberty, but in many cases they are children born with ambiguous external sexual characteristics, or men whose testicles have not descended. For convenience, transsexuals and transvestites are also lumped together with them. They live partly from alms that they receive for dancing at parties. In 2006 the Indian authorities deliberately employed a group of eunuchs to sing outside the houses of tax-evaders, with the object of embarrassing the offenders so acutely with their singing that they would finally pay up. According to the Indian press the campaign was very successful in the city of Patna in the eastern state of Bihar, where singing eunuchs collected over 7,000 euros.

As long ago as 1887 the British Governor-General promulgated a law forbidding castration, but the eunuchs are still there, not only in India, but also in Pakistan and Bangladesh. Most probably they are of Muslim origin, as indicated, for example, by the fact that they bury rather than cremate their dead. Most eunuchs live communally as *hijra* (meaning 'the third gender'), sharing their lot with transsexuals and transvestites. They play a part in certain rituals, or work as artists or healers, besides acting as singers or dancers at festivals marking births and marriages. The words of their songs are usually humorous and with a sexual tinge.

From time immemorial eunuchs have made a pilgrimage to the temple of Bechraji, about 100 km west of Ahmedabad, which houses the goddess Bahuchara-Mata. This goddess is associated with sexual abstinence and genital mutilation. According to legend a king once prayed to the goddess for a son. The son arrived, but when he became a man proved to be impotent. Bahuchara appeared to the man in a dream and asked him to serve her by cutting off his genitalia and donning women's clothes. The man did as the goddess asked and since then *hijras* have been supposed to hear a call from the gods in their sleep to divest themselves of their external sex organs. Even today there are always eunuchs to be found at a certain spot in the back garden of the temple in Bechraji, but they are not allowed inside. It is still said that when a baby boy is born with underdeveloped genitals he is taken to the temple by his family. The eunuchs receive the child and perform a simple ritual operation, followed by six weeks' seclusion, after which the child can become an apprentice *hijra*.

Ancient Rome

In Ancient Rome castration was a well-known phenomenon. At a later period, though the Church of Rome was not well disposed towards genitalia, a practice survived until 1913 of feeling between the legs of the candidate elected pope by the conclave of cardinals before he was allowed to mount the throne of St Peter – to make sure he was really a man. Any Catholic also knows that there is a hole in the seat of the Holy Chair. After all, in the past the cardinals had slipped up. In 855 they elected a certain Johanna, and that must not be allowed to happen a second time. Once one of the cardinals had confirmed the candidate's masculinity *de visu et tacto* (by sight and touch) through the hole in the chair, he pronounced the customary words 'Testiculos habet et bene pendentes' (He has testicles and they hang well). The cardinals then sang: 'Habet ova noster papa!' (Our pope has balls). Like the pope, candidate monks were closely examined for any abnormalities in those bodily parts, which they would subsequently be forbidden to use . . .

The Ancient Romans distinguished four different types: the true castrati, where both testicles and the penis had been removed, the *spadones*, who had lost only their testicles, the *thlibiae*, whose testicles had been destroyed by crushing and the *thlasiae* in whom only the seminal cords had been severed. Eventually castration took place on such a large scale that the emperor felt compelled to ban it. It was not doctors, but barbers or bath house attendants who carried out the procedure, and they were paid by slave traders and brothel-keepers, who initially had a monopoly. After the ban certain priests (of Cybele) continued to mutilate themselves – and not only themselves, but also any unfortunate youths who fell into their hands. They were called *galli*, or capons, and were destined to work as prostitutes.

In the Byzantine Empire it was also known that castrated men were less competitive and aggressive than men with testicles, which is why they were appointed as civil servants. One could take them at their word and they did what they were instructed to do, they knew they place and did not constitute a threat to the emperor and his followers.

Daniel and Potiphar

In several places in the Bible there is mention, sometimes in veiled terms, sometimes explicit, of castration and eunuchs. The Talmud is much clearer, for example about Daniel and his friends. In the Christian tradition Daniel is one of the great four: Isaiah, Jeremiah, Ezechiel and Daniel. In the book of Daniel the story is told of how the king of Babylon (Nebuchadnezzar) conquers Jerusalem and deports the Jews. In Babel Nebuchadnezzar orders his steward to select a number of strong young men for a three-year period of training as counsellors. In the Bible the head of the household is also called the head of the eunuchs, and in the Talmud it is stated that Daniel and his friends themselves became eunuchs. There is a great divergence of opinion among rabbis on the how and why. There is a story that Daniel and his friends were accused of immoral conduct before Nebuchadnezzar and, in order to defend themselves against this charge, they mutilated 'certain parts of their bodies' (meaning their sex organs) in order to prove that the accusations were groundless, so becoming eunuchs at their own instigation. Another commentator tells how Daniel mutilated himself in order not to have to marry a non-Jewish princess.

The most current view is that Daniel and his friends were castrated by the king's servants, so that they were no longer a danger to the women of the court. In addition, they were extremely useful to the king. Daniel was brilliant at explaining and interpreting dreams. No one could match him, and he was worth ten of any of the native diviners and exorcists.

By far the most famous eunuch in the Bible is Potiphar, who features in a classic story, with his wife. Joseph, the son of the patriarch Jacob and his wife Rachel, had been thrown into a well by his jealous brothers and subsequently sold to merchants. He was taken to Egypt, where he was resold to a courtier of the pharaoh called Potiphar. Potiphar was head of the bodyguards of Pharaoh Apepi II – in those days a most responsible and prominent position. There was an important precondition for those who came so close to the pharaoh: they must be castrated . . . Potiphar probably lived in the city of On, northeast of present-day Cairo, at the beginning of the Nile delta. At that time it was the scientific and religious heart of Egypt. Because it was the centre of sun-worship, and the Greeks later called it Heliopolis, the city of the sun.

Genesis tells us that God was with Joseph, so that he prospered. God's blessing followed him to the house of the Egyptian and it was not long before Joseph had risen to become Potiphar's closest assistant. He became overseer, administrator, butler and steward combined. Potiphar came to trust Joseph so implicitly that he put him in charge of all his possessions and henceforth concentrated solely on wining and dining.

One has to admit that Joseph had all the personal qualities imaginable. He was handsome and well built, intelligent and successful. Apart from that, in Ancient Egypt Syrian slaves were considered the best and Joseph was of Syrian (Aramaic) origin on both his father's and his mother's side. Syrians were preferred because the Egyptian ruling class belonged to the Hyksos, people who originated from Syria. There was also something mysterious about Joseph, so it was no wonder that he was noticed, especially by his master's wife: Joseph's presence brought excitement into her sexually dull life and his charms gradually became irresistible. Her invitation ('Come lie with me'), was therefore not long in coming. Joseph, however, refused: 'Behold, my master wotteth not what is with me in the house, and he hath committed all that he hath to my hand; there is none greater in this house than I; neither hath he kept back any thing from me but thee, because thou art his wife' (Genesis 39). Potiphar's wife was not impressed by this Salvation Army-style moral rectitude. Of course she persisted but her passion remained unrequited, since he was in the house day after day and continued to refuse.

One day she saw her chance: they were alone in the house. It was now or never. She went to him, clutched his robe and for the umpteenth time repeated her imperious question: 'Come lie with me.' Joseph tore himself free, leaving his garment in her hands. Her feelings turned to hate. She called her servants and said: 'See, he hath brought in an Hebrew unto us to mock us; he came in unto me to lie with me, and I cried with a loud voice: and it came to pass, when he heard that I lifted up my voice and cried, that he left his garment with me, and fled, and got him out.'

In the Aramaic version the text has a more modern flavour: 'She threw the white of an egg on the bed, called the domestic staff and said:

"Look at the semen stains that man left – the Hebrew whom your master has brought into the house to mock at us.""

When Potiphar heard the news he was furious, had Joseph arrested and thrown into the pharaoh's jail on a charge of attempted rape, without even giving him a chance to defend himself.

Actually all the attention in this story is focused on Joseph, the ideal man, yet also a man not averse to power. 'Potiphar's wife illuminates both sides of Joseph's personality', was an interpretation I once heard a clergyman give. Her passion shows how attractive he was and his response to questions how he revered God, but still . . .

Potiphar's wife seems to be a marginal figure, also shown by the fact that the Bible gives her no name. At the beginning of the story she is called 'Potiphar's wife', but disappears anonymously. But however little attention she is given in the modern Bible story, she is given all the more in the Jewish tradition, and even has a name: Zuleika. Jewish accounts describe her inviting her girlfriends over and having Joseph serve them in order to show him off. Her friends were so bowled over by Joseph's appearance that their knives slipped and they cut their fingers. When she pretended to be surprised, her friends replied: 'How are we supposed to look at our hands when you show us such a divine looking man?' The theme of the spoiled, bored woman who conceives a burning passion for a younger servant, tries to seduce him and when she fails, falsely accuses him of rape, is a perennial one.

What makes Potiphar's wife so different from other 'bad' women in biblical stories? Tamar, it's true, seduced her father-in-law, which is certainly not very edifying, but Potiphar's wife had completely different motives. She was used to the luxury of the high life, but was at the same time neglected, since Potiphar paid no attention to her. What she was looking for was distraction, or rather, simple sexual satisfaction. What she was hoping for was a fling, a one-night stand, that was all. 'And what was wrong with that?' I can still hear that country clergyman saying.

In the fourth century, in the sect of the Obelites, some men had themselves castrated on the basis of a text from the Bible (Matthew 19:12). Oddly enough they did not disapprove of marriage itself, but of sexual intercourse. Two centuries previously in the Near East a Gnostic sect, the Adamites, had emerged, whose aim was to invoke heaven by the suppression of all sensual desires: in imitation of Adam they went around naked in their religious observances. These strange excrescences undoubtedly spring from early Christian thinking on martyrdom and the accompanying physical abstinence, self-chastisement and privations as the only way to salvation. Castration was condemned as early as 323, at the Council of Nicaea, and the ordination of eunuchs was forbidden. In forbidding (self-)castration and excluding castrati from the priesthood Christianity became more Roman, since in the Eastern Church particularly castrated priests like Cybele and Attis were revered. Many castrated monks and bishops were active in the Byzantine Christian church. Until the late Middle Ages eunuchs were even appointed bishops in the Eastern Church, among them Theophylactus, an eleventh-century bishop of Bulgaria, whose seat was in Ochrida.

The French philosopher Pierre Abélard (1079–1142) believed that the mutilation of his own genitalia had been appointed by God and that castration would make him a better theologian.

The Skoptsy

Much later, in the eighteenth century, in the Russian Skoptsy sect, it became the custom after fathering two children to have not just the testicles but the greater part of the penis removed. First the testicles were destroyed (originally with red-hot iron bars, but later a knife was preferred). The second procedure comprised the removal of the penis. After the first stage the result was referred to as 'The Minor Seal' and after the second as 'The Great Seal'. Seal is a concept that features extensively in the impenetrable Book of Revelation. After castration there was an interval of several years before the penis was removed, which may be the reason why, according to the records, no serious complications occurred. The Skoptsy regarded the testicles as the keys to hell. Removal gave them the right to remount 'the pale horse', undoubtedly a reference to passages from Revelation, 6:

> And when he had opened the fourth seal, I heard the voice of
> the fourth beast say, Come and see. And I looked and behold
> a pale horse: and his name that sat on him was Death, and Hell
> followed with him. And power was given to them over the
> fourth part of the earth, to kill with sword, and with hunger,
> and with death, and with the beasts of the earth.

The penis too, then, was simply the key to hell. In her fascinating book on the sect (*Castration and the Heavenly Kingdom*) Laura Engelstein shows that the hell was of course a metaphor for the vagina.

After cutting off the penis the person conducting the operation would say a prayer and cry out: 'The Lord has truly risen!' The castrato was now ready to mount the pale horse:

> And I saw when the Lamb opened one of the seals, and I heard,
> as it were the noise of thunder, one of the four beasts saying,

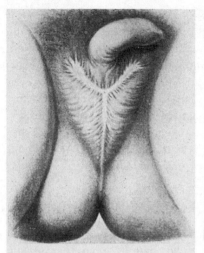 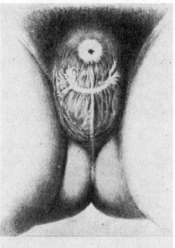

'The Minor Seal' and 'The Great Seal'.

Come and see. And I saw, and behold a white horse: and he that sat on him had a bow; and crown was given unto him: and he went forth conquering, and to conquer. [Revelations 6]

To make urinating possible after the operation, though, the follower concerned did temporarily require a tin or lead tube in his urethra.

Female members of the sect did not damage their ovaries, but did mutilate their labia, clitoris, breasts and nipples.

The sect originated from a group of flagellants, which included a certain Andrey Ivanov. He and his followers wanted to take a stand against the Klysty family, who had been accused of licentiousness, and founded the Skoptsy sect, after the Russian word *skopets*, eunuch. The sect rejects most of the dogmas of the Russian Orthodox Church, specifically redemption by Jesus Christ on the cross. The sect preached castration as salvation, basing themselves mainly on passages from Isaiah 56:

Neither let the eunuch say, Behold I am a dry tree. For thus saith the Lord unto the eunuchs that keep my Sabbaths, and choose the things that please me, and take hold of my covenant; even unto them will I give in mine house and within my walls a place and a name better than of sons and daughters: I will give them an everlasting name that shall not be cut off.

These eunuchs could no longer have sons and daughters, but God promised them something better than the transience of descendants.

The founder of the Skoptsy, Andrey Ivanov, met a less glorious fate. He was arrested and deported to Siberia, and the leadership passed to Kondrati Selivanov, one of his first followers. Selivanov later preached in St Petersburg under the protection of Baroness von Krüdener, one of the Czar's mistresses, who regarded the preacher as a saint.

The Skoptsy denied themselves not only sexual pleasure, but also parties, gambling and alcohol. Meanwhile many bankers and money-lenders were converted, which might explain why many members of the sect became millionaires, using their wealth mainly to propagate their ideology. For me, the story of the Skoptsy echoes that of the Church of Scientology, with its celebrity converts such as Tom Cruise. At its height the sect is thought to have had almost 150,000 members, but it was struck a severe blow in 1917 when the Bolsheviks passed antireligious legislation and there was widespread persecution. In 1929 a big anti-Skoptsy trial was held in Leningrad, and many sect members sought asylum in Romania, where there was still freedom of religion.

Two octaves higher

In the seventeenth and eighteenth centuries not only the directors of opera companies, but also the Catholic Church made grateful use of men castrated at a young age. In Italy at that time, if you had a reasonable voice when you were ten and came from a poor family there was a good chance that you would be recruited, with the local priest acting as a go-between. That meant being crudely castrated before your voice broke: your testicles were plunged into boiling water, causing them to shrivel. The Adam's apple did not develop, though the rest of the body did, and in this way the effect of the voice breaking was prevented once and for all. In addition, after puberty the castrato would have a small larynx over an ample ribcage; this could of course be filled with large amounts of air, which he could then force out through his relatively small glottal apertures. The men retained their high-pitched voices and could continue to sing soprano roles into adulthood.

Both the parents and the boy were tempted with the prospect of free training as an opera singer and the accompanying singing career. But what is true now was just as true then: 'for many be called, but few chosen' (Matthew 20:16). An opera career or a permanent position as a singer in the Sistine Chapel was something only a few could aspire to. If someone failed to make the big time, a relatively meagre existence as a priest or something similar beckoned. What was the cost to the castrated boy? All his life he would have a tendency to obesity, his penis would remain small and no seminal glands would develop. He would not develop the normal male pattern of hair growth, but nor would he go bald. And however long he lay in the sun, he would never tan.

There are various explanations of exactly how and why castrati came into being. The most logical answer is that at that time women were forbidden to appear on stage, and female roles were taken by castrati. Another explanation is that the castrato embodies the trinity of male and female lust and childlike beauty. This view links to the Ancient Greek androgynous ideal: the uniting of the male and the female. The castrati were the pop stars of their age. If a castrato struck it rich, he could achieve an almost divine status. In Italy a successful castrato voice was called a *canaro elefante*, a canary's voice in the body of an elephant.

The 1994 film *Farinelli* gives a romanticized picture of a famous castrato. The film's subject is Carlo Broschi (1705–1782), stage name Farinelli, one of the most famous Italian castrati, who also played keyboard instruments and occasionally composed and wrote lyrics. Broschi was castrated at about the age of seven. He was an exception to the rule that most castrati were of humble origin: his father was a nobleman and governor of Apulia. He was sent to a music school founded especially for castrati, where he developed his voice under the direction of Nicola Porpora. He became known in Southern Italy as *Il Ragazzo* (The Boy). In 1720 Farinelli sang in public for the first time, performing a piece by his mentor. Two years later he made his debut in Rome, where the audience was particularly enthusiastic about his ability to sustain notes of great purity. He toured all through Europe, and a Milanese critic wrote of him: 'Farinelli had a piercing, full, rich, clear and well-modulated soprano voice, with a range from A below middle C to D three octaves above middle C. His intonation was pure, his breath-control exceptional and he had a very flexible throat, so that he could execute the longest intervals quickly and with the greatest of ease.'

In 1724 he visited London and appeared in *Artaserse*, a work for which his brother had written most of the music. The Prince of Wales and the whole court showered him with compliments and gifts. After three years in England, he left for Spain, stopping en route for a few months in France, where he sang for Louis XIV. His original intention was to spend only a few months in Spain, but it eventually became almost 25 years. The queen used Farinelli's voice to cure her husband, Philip V, of his pathological melancholy. The singer became as powerful as any minister, but was wise enough to use that power very discreetly. For two decades Farinelli sang songs evening after evening for the depressed king. After the succession of Ferdinand V, Farinelli was appointed theatre director in Madrid and Aranjuez. In 1750 the

Alessandro
Moreschi.

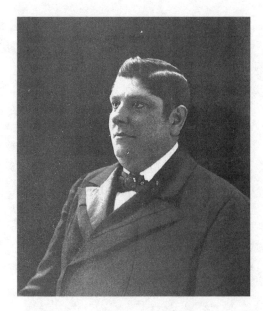

castrato was knighted, but when Charles III ascended the throne
Farinelli returned to Italy, where he spent the rest of his life.

The most sensational stories circulated about the sexual dissipation of castrati: they were sterile, but by no means always impotent. In
addition they had a certain tenderness about them, an attractive combination for women in an age without contraceptives.

Sadly there is only one recording of a man castrated as a pre-
adolescent: it dates from the beginning of the twentieth century, and the
recording is probably not representative, since the singer, Alessandro
Moreschi, was already advanced in years and was certainly not a top-
flight singer.

Legal action against men without balls

The Church Father St Augustine (354–430) had already stated that in
sexual relations there should always be the hope of fertilization. And
in the past at least that was only possible with a stiff penis and normal
testicles. 'Go forth and multiply,' as it says in Genesis. Well, impotent
men were incapable of that and hence were violating the sacrament of
marriage – it was as simple as that. From the thirteenth century
onwards, following Augustine, ecclesiastical law considered it more or
less a mortal sin if impotent and hence infertile men turned out to
have entered into marriage. The same applied to eunuchs and hermaphrodites and men with undescended testicles, who for that reason
could be indicted by an ecclesiastical court.

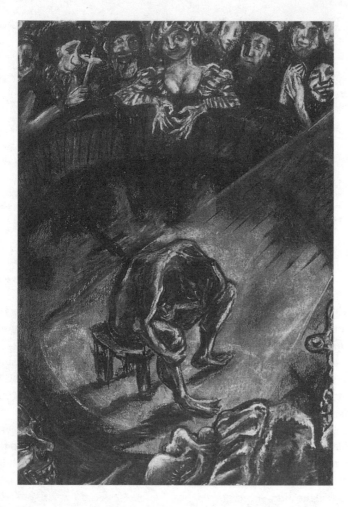

A public erection.

During the trial the defendants in any case had to prove that they possessed a normal sexual apparatus, and a jury composed of theologians, doctors and midwives had to assess it. From the trial proceedings it is clear that where necessary the jurors even spent the night at the defendant's bedside in order to be able to judge any nocturnal erections occurring. The pompous rituals surrounding these trials indirectly confirmed the power of the Catholic Church. Originally there was a degree of discretion, but during the course of the sixteenth century the church authorities made the leap from mental to actual voyeurism. Not only was a demonstration of the erect member required, but its 'elasticity and natural movement' must be demonstrated. Sometimes the jury even demanded 'a proof of ejaculation'. Naturally this was eventually no longer sufficient and the married couple had to make love in the presence of the jury, the so-called congress.

The treatment of eunuchs and hermaphrodites also showed that for the church there was a taboo on pleasure. Though eunuchs could not ejaculate, some of them could manage a quite satisfactory erection, so that their wives were by no means always unsatisfied. But after 1587, irrespective of the wishes of the partners, these marriages had to be annulled by decree of Pope Sixtus V. This gruesome pope could not bear to think that these men should sleep in the same bed as their wives instead of living chastely together. He wrote about this in a letter to the papal nuncio in Spain, who was also bishop of Navarre. According to Sixtus, the eunuchs had consorted with women 'with filthy lewdness' and 'impure embraces' and even presumed to have a right to marry. In the pope's eyes the fact that the women knew of this 'defect' made the offence all the more grave. Sixtus was taking to its logical conclusion both Augustine and Thomas Aquinas' view of procreation as the primal and true goal of marriage.

In Greek mythology Hermaphroditus was the son of the gods Hermes and Aphrodite. On one of his journeys the nymph Salmacis falls in love with him because of his great physical beauty. She tries to seduce him, but fails. When he goes for a swim in a cool lake, believing himself alone, Salmacis dives in after him, and embraces and kisses him. She prays to the gods that she may be united with him. Her prayer is answered, and they become one flesh.

In the seventeenth and eighteenth centuries French society was caught up in a furious public debate on the differences between men and women. In his book *Damning the Innocent* the French historian Pierre Darmon states that there was a certain envy of the supposedly unbridled sex lives of deviants. From the sixteenth century onwards hermaphrodites – who during the Middle Ages were sometimes burned alive and were regarded as children of Satan – received an apparently milder treatment. They were examined by doctors and midwives, who subsequently stated publicly which sex was applicable. In doubtful cases the person involved was allowed to choose for himself/herself, but then had to abide by that choice for the rest of his/her life. Leaving one's sexual role open or occasionally switching identities, as the mood took one, as Marie/Marin le Marcis tried to do, was unforgivable fraud. This hermaphrodite chambermaid fell in love with a fellow maid, decided it was more useful to go through life as a man from then on and married her, with her full consent. To their astonishment the happy young pair were immediately detained, imprisoned and brought before the court. The experts unanimously accused them of fraud and, inevitably, sodomy and obscenity. 'If one of the jury had not ventured to feel Marin's private parts – and felt something masculine – the poor man would have been burnt alive and his wife flogged in the market place and afterwards banished.' As it was things turned out differently: Marin was reprieved, but was condemned to live as a woman.

An angel with balls

In 1908 the avant-garde sculptor Jacob Epstein designed an angel for the tomb of Oscar Wilde in the cemetery of Père Lachaise in Paris. 'Homosexuals, artists and writers are outcasts' reads the verse inscription. Epstein's angel was not placed on the grave without a fight. There was a great commotion among all involved about the dimensions of its testicles. They were unusually large, it was maintained in a meeting. However, that would not have been difficult, since according to the Judaeo-

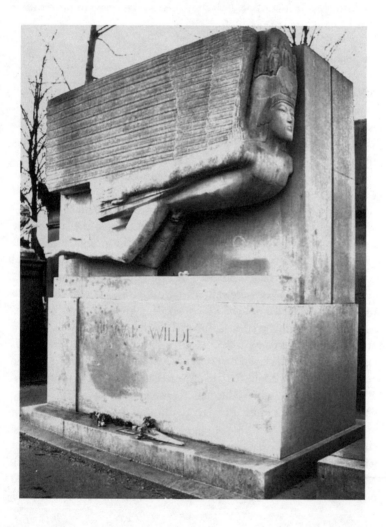

The grave of
Oscar Wilde.

Christian norm, angels should not have any testicles at all, being sexless. The sex of the angel was probably a homage to Oscar Wilde by Epstein.

Whatever the considerations of the moralizers of Père Lachaise may have been, a consensus soon emerged on what should be done with the angel: either castration or a chaste fig leaf. Pending a final decision it was hidden from view by a tarpaulin. Much later the angel, now once again on view naked and intact, became a place of pilgrimage for gays. So many visitors gave the balls a quick stroke that they acquired a patina, their shiny surface standing out against the matt white sculpture. Until in 1963 things went wrong. Two British ladies, who had taken offence at the angel's balls, hatched a plan. They paid the angel a second visit armed with hammer and chisel. Looking around furtively, they chipped the balls off. The action of the prim ladies had little to do with climbing up the hierarchy. A gardener found the angel's testicles on the ground near the grave and took them to the superintendent, who found a use for them as paperweights.

Eunuchs in the twenty-first century

In the United States an estimated 40,000 men per year are chemically castrated as a treatment for metastasized prostate cancer. In many cases the growth of this type of cancer is dependent on testosterone, at least in the initial phase. In the Netherlands 7,000 new patients are diagnosed with prostate cancer each year. Until well into the 1980s the castration was performed surgically, which was certainly no joke for the patients involved. True, they were mostly older men, but even so . . . Nowadays the procedure is carried out chemically, usually with prolonged-release depot injections in the abdominal wall. The injections consist of gonadorelins, or LH-RH analogues. LH-RH stands for luteinizing hormone-releasing hormone. These medicines act mainly on the brain (hypothalamushypophysis). Examples include Suprefact 9.45 mg injection, Zoladex 10.8 mg injection, Lucrin 11.25 mg and Decapeptyl 3.75 mg.

The most frequent side-effects are tiredness and headache. Hair growth also decreases, and the hair becomes softer. Approximately 5 per cent of testosterone production takes places in the adrenal glands. In order to shut down production completely, so-called antiandrogens can be given in addition. These include Androcur 50 mg (250–300 mg per day), Anandron 300 mg (150–300 mg per day), Flutamide 250 mg (750 mg per day) and Casodex 50 mg (50 mg per day). One of the most troublesome side-effects of these drugs is painful breast formation. This can be prevented by one-off radiation treatment of a small area around both nipples.

When the patient starts on a course of an LH-RH analogue an additional dose of an antiandrogen is given in order to prevent a flare-up of the disease due to stimulation of the hypophysis and the resultant rise in testosterone production. After four weeks the gland is saturated with LH-RH analogue and hence the production of testosterone is blocked. Long-term treatment with an LH-RH analogue plus an antiandrogen is called a 'total' androgen treatment. This is mostly used in men with metastasized prostate cancer. Hormonal treatment of metastatized prostate cancer is effective in between 70 and 80 per cent of cases.

The average time lapse between the start of the hormonal treatment and the emergence of a hormone-resistant illness, is between a year and a half and two years, meaning that after that time the hormonal treatment no longer has sufficient effect. Although the usefulness of continuing treatment with an LH-RH compound in the case of hormone-resistant prostate cancer has not been incontrovertibly established, the experts believe that when the cancer worsens during treatment with an LH-RH analogue it is better to continue the therapy. This avoids the eventuality that besides the hormone-resistant prostate cancer cells there is a resurgence in the growth of cancer cells still sensitive to (and hence inhibited by) the hormonal treatment. Although there is no conclusive proof, there are strong indications for the correctness of this assumption, since it was shown by research in the 1990s that the period of patient survival was shorter when the hormone treatment had been terminated, compared with patients with whom the treatment had been continued. This is why even in cases where chemotherapy is given, treatment with an LH-RH is in fact continued. Even in the case of chemical castration – as the name implies, not much is left of the testicles. Prostate cancer patients in effect become eunuchs.

chapter six

Ailments of the Scrotum

As long ago as the nineteenth century it was known that certain medicines could damage the testicles. Félix Roubaud, a famous French physician, described how in treating tuberculosis with iodine vapours he had observed four cases of progressive sexual impotence. He found 'a marked wasting of the testicles'. Saltpetre was also found to be harmful, the use of bromide compounds affected mainly sexual desire, while camphor inhibited the 'sensitivity of the sexual system'. Nowadays it is anti-cancer medication in particular that has a bad name in this respect. Other drugs that can adversely affect the production of sperm cells are salazopyrine (used for inflammation of the intestine), indomethacine (rheumatism), ranitidine and cimetidine (stomach complaints), nitrofurantoine (urinary tract infections), spironolacton (a diuretic), allopurinol (gout), cyclosporine (an anti-rejection agent in transplants) and various hormonal preparations. Gossypol is a natural component of cotton seed oil, which in some parts of China is used in the kitchen. Strikingly, in those regions male fertility was clearly reduced. The Chinese plant *Tryptergium wilfordii* can also cause reduced fertility.

As mentioned in the previous chapter, men with metastatized prostate cancer are mostly given medication to reduce testosterone to what is called 'castration level' (surgical castration is scarcely if ever carried out today). Even for elderly men this remains quite an onerous procedure. Partly because of their often advanced age most prostate cancer patients are no longer able to achieve a firm and lasting erection. The hormonal therapy results in hot flushes, comparable with menopausal symptoms in women. In addition there is the risk of osteoporosis and the accompanying increased danger of fractures.

Erotic fantasies are stimulated by testosterone, and therefore one would expect them to peter out. But that is by no means always the case: the memory has stored many of these fantasies. This phenomenon is sometimes called *cinema érotique intérieur*. In such cases erotic caresses by an understanding partner can therefore do wonders. No one should underestimate the fulfilment and satisfaction this can bring, particularly in old men close to death. Knowing one is suffering from incurable prostate cancer and still feeling some life in one's sexual organs can provide a much-needed boost.

Alcohol has a toxic effect on the functioning of the testicles, and in the case of chronic abuse less testosterone is produced and the liver is less and less capable of breaking down oestrogen (men produce small quantities of this female hormone). In contrast to men, in women sexual excitement usually increases under the influence of alcohol. Why is that?

In both sexes sexual interest and sexual arousal are related to the testosterone level in the blood. But with women things are more complicated: in their case the production of the male sex hormone (in the adrenal gland, in fat tissue and in the ovaries) varies with the menstrual cycle: the testosterone level is highest in the fertile period around ovulation. Researchers have discovered that a relatively small amount of alcohol (two glasses of beer or wine) is sufficient to cause the testosterone level to rise. The effect is found only around ovulation if no contraceptive pill is used. In the case of women who stop taking the pill the effect is all the greater because with the contraceptive pill the testosterone level remains relatively low throughout the cycle.

Self-examination

A man who wants to know exactly how things are put together down in his scrotum can find out most easily by sitting in a hot bath and feeling himself. Besides being informative, such a voyage of discovery can help in identifying any abnormality at an early date, assuming of course that one has some knowledge of the anatomy of the scrotum. The surface of a healthy testicle feels smooth, with no irregularities. Distinguishing the testicle itself and the epididymis is fairly simple: the epididymis hangs behind the testicle like a runner bean. At the bottom, where its tail begins the epididymis merges with the seminal duct; this can also be easily located and felt.

The chance that in the course of such a self-examination one will find a lump between one's thumb and forefinger that according to the textbooks shouldn't be there, is quite high. However, this should not lead to immediate panic, since in the great majority of cases this is fluid. The best-known forms of this are the *spermatocele*, filled with a grey liquid which under microscopic examination reveals sperm cells, the *hydrocele*, filled with pale yellow-coloured clear liquid, and the *hematocele*, filled with blood.

Undescended testicles

A ridgeling stallion is one in which both testicles have remained at the back of the abdominal cavity and have not descended into the scrotum. Such horses are almost always infertile. With mares, however, he behaves just like a normal stallion, since he still produces normal quantities of testosterone. If the animal is sold as a gelding, the new owner may experience problems, as a ridgeling stallion is inevitably less placid than a gelding. In this way undescended testicles can lead to great confusion and dissension.

In Ancient Rome men with two undescended testicles were not allowed to appear in court as witnesses. Roughly speaking, 20 per cent of cases involved two undescended testicles. The Ancient world did have some notion of surgery, but the range of operations was limited. In fact in those days the choice was between being castrated brutally or with a razor-sharp knife. Moving undescended testicles to their appointed place was impossible. There is little point in treating undescended testicles with medication in the form of hormones and this is scarcely ever done these days. Too often hormones proved ineffective and an operation was subsequently needed anyway.

Over 80 per cent of undescended testicles can be seen or felt in the groin. If they can be neither felt nor seen, doctors speak of cryptoorchidism, meaning literally 'hidden testicle'. That usually means that the testicle has got stuck somewhere behind the abdominal cavity. These make up some 20 per cent of the total. Tissue examination of undescended testicles shows irreversible abnormalities in the sperm-cell producing tissue from six months after birth onwards. It is therefore crucial to relocate the testicle as soon as possible, that is, in the scrotum. This kind of procedure is called *orchidopexy*, and in it the testicle is inserted and secured in the scrotum. If the seminal cord is short this can be a particularly awkward operation.

Cryptoorchidism is also found in animals. In cats the abnormality is fairly rare (0.7%), but in dogs it occurs regularly (between 0.8% and 11%, depending on the breed). It is most common in small breeds such as poodles, Yorkshire terriers, dachshunds, Chihuahuas, Maltese terriers, toy schnauzers and shelties. Dogs with this abnormality are excluded from breeding. As in humans, if left untreated the sperm quality is anyway exceptionally poor. There are some animals in which cryptoorchidism is normal. In almost all marine mammals, with their streamlined shape, the testicles are located in the abdominal cavity, and the same applies to elephants and hippopotami.

In humans, if the testicle cannot be felt, keyhole surgery is first carried out to check whether the testicle has been formed at all. If the testicle is located high up behind the abdominal cavity, the distance is too great to bring it down together with its stalk. In that case a clamp is put on the stalk, that is, on the artery and vein, after which the blood supply is taken over by the small artery belonging to the seminal duct. This is followed six months later by a second procedure in order to transfer the testicle to the scrotum, a procedure which can also be performed by keyhole surgery.

Being born with a testicle lodged behind the abdomen involves an increased risk of testicular cancer, which is not decreased by timely relocation in the scrotum. In addition it quite frequently happens that no connection is found between such a testicle and the epididymis, which of course means that no sperm cells can be expected from the testicle concerned. It is important in all cases to pinpoint the position of both testicles on the 'testicular map' immediately after birth. It is highly improbable that a testicle which has first been located in the scrotum will move to a position behind the abdominal cavity. The 'testicular map' is important in the diagnosis of a 'retractile testicle'. For a short period after birth the previously explained cremaster reflex is not yet present. The reflex goes on increasing until puberty, quite frequently causing boys' testicles to be pulled into the groin. If there is no 'testicular map' and there is doubt whether the diagnosis should be 'undescended testicle' or 'retractile testicle', it sometimes helps to examine the child while he is lying in a warm bath or squatting.

Multiple testicles

Men with no testicles, one testicle or two are nothing out of the ordinary, but men with three are rare. A story is told of a monk who was unable to keep his vow of chastity because of having three testicles, while an eighteenth-century account describes a man with multiple testicles, a condition known medically as *polyorchidy*, who was capable of sexual intercourse up to his hundred and twenty-fifth year. Others were reputedly capable of ejaculating twenty times in one night. Ambrosius Paré, one of the giants of medical history, believed that extra testicles were a common phenomenon, and many surgeons shared his view. Undoubtedly these were almost always spermatoceles that were mistaken for additional testicles.

In a medical career of nearly thirty years I have only ever encountered one case of multiple testicles. The boy in question had three – a case of *triorchidy*, which can take various forms. There may be an extra testicle without an epididymis or seminal duct (a), an extra testicle with an epididymis but without a seminal duct (b), an extra testicle with an epididymis attached to the seminal duct of a testicle located below (c),

The various
forms of poly-
orchidy.

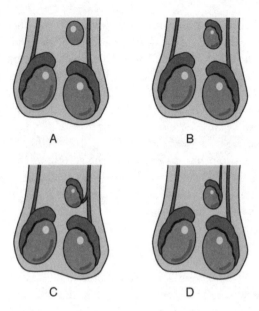

A   B

C   D

and an extra testicle with an epididymis and an extra seminal duct. These are different kinds of tissue faults between the sixth and eighth week in the development of the embryo, the period during which it is decided whether one is going to look like a girl or a boy as regards external sexual characteristics.

Most patients with polyorchidy present with a painless swelling. The most common location for the abnormality is on the left. In most men the diagnosis is made between the ages of fifteen and 25, and in 80 per cent of cases tissue examination of removed additional testicles showed a reduced or non-existent production of sperm cells. M. Hakami and S. H. Mosavy described a man with fertile sperm in whom the third testicle was discovered only after a vasectomy on both sides.

Inguinal hernia

The testicles are formed at the spot where the kidneys are situated, high up behind the abdominal cavity. From there they descend through the inguinal canal into the scrotum. On that journey – the baby boy is still in his mother's womb – they take the front of the abdominal membrane with them. When things proceed normally this bulge in the abdominal membrane closes, so that there is no open connection left with the abdominal cavity. The remnant of abdominal membrane in the scrotum surrounds the testicles for the rest of the individual's life as a double-layered protective membrane.

If that hernial sac does not close around birth, then there is a chance that the intestine of the newborn infant will descend as far as the scrotum, creating a so-called innate hernia, which sometimes manifests itself as a sizeable swelling. Of course a hernia requires surgery – in boys with a scalpel, in adults mostly by means of keyhole surgery. Adults in whom the abdominal membrane has closed properly may suffer a hernia because of an increase in pressure due, for example, to chronic coughing or a great deal of heavy lifting. Often the intestines bulge into the groin but do not reach the scrotum. The doctor can ascertain whether there is a hernia by having the man blow against the back of his hand while standing and himself feeling the inguinal canal with his finger from the scrotum.

Torsio testis

Acute, intense pain on one side of the scrotum indicates a twisted stalk (*torsio*) of the *testis*. This seems to happen to one man in 4,000 annually. The testicles do not lie loose in the scrotum: they are attached to it by a wide band which prevents the testicle from turning vertically on its axis. There are some men, mostly aged between ten and 30, in whom the band is too long and often too narrow. One day they may have the unfortunate experience of one of their testicles starting to turn: this is impossible to mistake, since the victim feels sudden intense pain in the scrotum, spilling over into the groin. The scrotum becomes red or purple, and patient is often nauseous. In a physical examination the observant doctor will notice in a case of torsion the cremaster reflex, the retraction of the testicles in the direction of the groin when the inside of the thigh is stroked. It can happen that a torsion disappears spontaneously after a short time, and with it the pain. Even then it is advisable to consult a doctor, since the phenomenon will undoubtedly recur one day, and it's doubtful whether expert help will be on hand.

The fact is that *torsio testis* can have unpleasant consequences. As a result of the twisting of the testicle pressure is put on the veins and the artery. The flow of blood is interrupted and, if the situation continues for more than a few hours, the tissue in the testicle will die off for want of oxygen. The speed with which that happens depends on the extent to which the testicle has turned on its own axis. Sometimes it may have turned 360 degrees, in which case the process will be very rapid. The sperm-producing cells particularly are sensitive to a lack of oxygen, while those that make testosterone, the Leydig cells, survive longer. If a twisted testicle is untwisted within about four hours there need be no further repercussions. This need not, by the way, require an operation; an expert doctor may in the first instance attempt to solve the problem manually. He or she should keep in mind the image of a heavy book, say a massive King James Bible, which has to be opened – outwards.

Occasionally a *torsio testis* is not recognized and the pain and swelling are attributed to an inflammation of the epididymis, so subsequently a completely wrong treatment is applied, usually with antibiotics. This results in the completely unnecessary loss of an important organ. When in doubt, the best thing to do is to operate immediately, possibly after a duplex echograph. In this kind of operation the other testicle is immediately included, that is stabilized, to ensure that the problem will never be repeated on that side.

Inflammation of the epididymis

Pain in the scrotum with a sudden onset and which is often intense can also be caused by *epididymitis*, or inflammation of the epididymis. This kind of caused is produced by a bacterium that has spread from the urinary tracts to the seminal duct and from there to the epididymis. Nowadays in younger people this is almost always *chlamydia trachomatis*, which is transmitted through sex. In the case of an inflammation of the epididymis, an extremely painful swelling develops at the back of the testicle, and soon afterwards the scrotum becomes hard and swollen. Anyone continuing to suffer in silence runs the risk of the testicle itself and hence fertility being affected. Inflammation of the epididymis is easy to treat with antibiotics, but if there is any doubt about the cause the GP will generally send his or her patient along for a urine culture to check what micro-organism has caused the inflammation of the urinary tracts. Experience shows that many men with an inflammation of the epididymis are not treated in time, or for long enough or with the wrong antibiotic, with the result that the infection may spread to the testicle itself, causing *epididymo-orchitis*. Complications include abcesses and the risk that after 'recovery' one is left with a 'shrivelled testicle'. It is also important that the patient rest as far as possible, and it is sensible to support the scrotum with a flannel containing ice, or an ice-pack.

Hydrocele

As has been said, after the closure of the hernial sac a remnant of the abdominal membrane carried along on the descent continues to surround each of the testicles as a double-layered sheet. Between those two layers there is normally a small quantity of liquid, which allows the testicle as it were to dance. Sometimes too much liquid is produced between the two layers, which can lead to a very large, uncomfortable

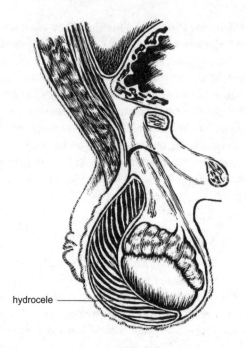

Hydrocele.

hydrocele

swelling called a hydrocele. If such a hernia becomes troublesome, for example, when cycling or during sexual intercourse, an operation is called for.

This cabaret song by Hans Dorrestein gives a humorous slant on hydroceles and sex:

Geriatric Sex

Sex for us wrinklies shows the wear and tear,
reflects the elderly wife.
God, when will he come, the poor old sod?
His prick's grown like a goat's hoof with no hair.
Sex for us wrinklies shows the wear and tear,
his scrotum's like a pouffe that's full of air.
After forty years it isn't odd,
growing as close as peas in a pod,
but when *this* is over I won't care,
sex for us wrinklies shows the wear and tear.

Hydrocele may be triggered by a previous inflammation of the epididymis, a trauma, or in vary rare cases testicular cancer, though in the majority of cases the cause remains obscure. It may be removed either via the groin or via the scrotum. In the latter case an incision is made in the skin and the next layer, the *tunica dartos*. Bleeding vessels are held with a fine pincette and cauterized. If the hydrocele is very large, it is first lanced and emptied by suction. The *tunica vaginalis* is cut open lengthways, so that the testicle itself can be taken out. The redundant layer is removed and folded back behind the epididymis. Because the wall of the hydrocele is turned inside out, the chance of relapse is small. Because of the abundant blood there is a high risk of bleeding after this operation, and partly because of this a pipe is frequently left in through which blood can drain away.

Spermatocele

The weird idea of 'growing an extra ball' is particularly common with spermatocele. This is because a hydrocele is as it were attached to the testicle, which as a result appears to grow bigger and bigger, while a spermatocele can be felt separately from the testicle, always at the level of the head of the epididymis. A weak spot may occur in the wall of the tubes between the testicle and the epididymis, a bulge develops and sperm cells accumulate in it. Such spermatoceles are very common: most middle-aged men have one or two. There are generally small, do not hurt and can do absolutely no harm. However, sometimes they grow to such proportions that it becomes difficult to go on walking with them. Anyone who consults a specialist and is told that an operation is proposed would be well advised to ask whether that operation is really necessary. There is a risk of damage to the artery to the testicle, inflammation and bleeding may occur, and moreover there is no guarantee that very shortly there will not be a recurrence of spermatocele. In order to prevent that the whole epididymis would have to be removed: with men who still want to have children it is completely disastrous to start operating.

Varicocele

To understand how a varicose vein or varicocele emerges it is necessary to know something about the blood supply to the testicles, or rather the drainage of blood. Venal blood leaves the testicles via the left and right testicular veins (*vena spermatica interna*). The right-hand vessel discharges into the inferior vena cava, which transports low-oxygen blood back to the heart. In the case of the left-hand testicular vein the situation is slightly different: it discharges into the left-hand renal vein, which transports blood purified in the left kidney to the vena cava. Since no organ, including a testicle, likes used blood, which contains waste matter, there are, especially in the left testicular vein, valves that prevent the blood from flowing back to the testicle. If those valves do not function properly it is possible that blood from the left renal artery will flow back, resulting in the formation of a varicose vein just above the left testicle, where there is a dense network of blood vessels (the *plexus pampiniformis*). This can lead to nagging pain, especially in men who stand up all day long. The accumulation of venal blood may cause the local temperature to rise, with possible harmful effects on fertility. But if the left testicle no longer functions properly, surely that won't affect the right one? You'd certainly think not, but in practice in a number of cases of varicose veins venal blood flows back on the right-hand side too. This is because there are communication channels between the left and right side, but gravity undoubtedly also plays a part, since varicose veins have never yet been observed in the scrotums of quadrupeds. Apart from that, varicose veins differ widely. Quite a few men, estimated at between 10 and 18 per hundred, have a varicose vein, but by no means everyone has a problem with it. Some 30 per cent of all men who consult a doctor because of involuntary childlessness have such a vein.

Making the diagnosis is generally quite simple. In half of patients the varicose vein is either visible to the naked eye or can be felt with the hand. In order to be able to assess the whole situation, the doctor will ask the patient to blow on the back of his hand briefly. A manoeuvre like this propels venal blood and causes the vein in the scrotum to swell considerably. If the doctor is not sure of his or her ground, he or she will ask for an ecograph of the scrotum. Surgery is by no means always called for in all cases of varicocele. With most men it is sufficient to advise the use of a tight-fitting pair of underpants. Only if the patient wishes to have children is treatment worthwhile. Researchers from Rotterdam showed recently in an excellent study that treating a varico-

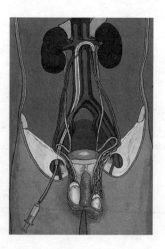

'Plugging' the left spermatic vein.

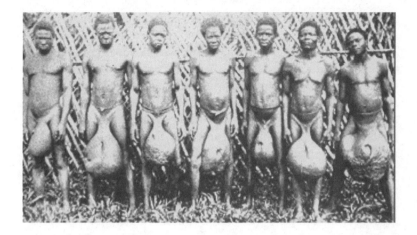

Scrotal lymphoedema resulting from filariasis.

cele significantly improves the chances of spontaneous pregnancy in the partner. There are three various possible treatments: surgically via an incision to the left of the navel, the groin or the scrotum, but also with an embolization in which a catheter is passed through the inguinal vein to the renal vein, after which a plug closure is inserted in the vena spermatica interna. The third possibility is a keyhole operation in which the vein is clipped. There is scarcely any difference between the success rates of the various treatments.

Lymphoedema

The scrotum can grow to an enormous size due to an accumulation of lymph. There are many underlying causes. One is the wearing of a clamp around the penis which passes behind the scrotum. This type of tourniquet does not generally lead to problems if continued for only a short time, and sometimes greatly adds to sexual pleasure.

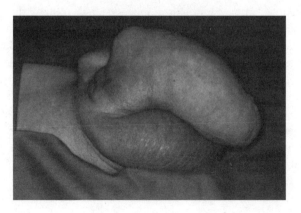

Lymphoedema of unknown origin.

Lymphoedema is caused by the accumulation of lymph in subcutaneous tissue. A Sanskrit book shows that treatments for lymphoedema of the penis and scrotum were practised as long ago as the third century BC. Worldwide the most common cause is filariasis. It is a disease in which the lymph canals become clogged by worms. Other causes include erysipelas, tuberculosis, syphilis, leprosy and cancer in the pelvis minor. Sometimes the cause is the total absence of any lymph vessels in that area: this is in fact an innate abnormality, the results of which usually manifest themselves only after the age of four.

There are various possible treatments, for example the use of diuretic pills, supporting bandages (cycling shorts are excellent), an operation to make connections between lymph vessels and veins, and best of all, the complete removal of the diseased tissue and the covering of the lower layers with skin grafts.

Injuries

According to George Gould and Walter Pyle in *Anomalies and Curiosities of Medicine*, ancient medical texts from India describe how women of the Cossiah tribe killed their husbands premeditatedly by grabbing their balls in a single movement and then squeezing as hard as possible until they dropped down dead. Not that long ago the author had to stitch a tear running lengthways across the scrotum of a man of about 40. Following a nocturnal row after excessive indulgence in alcohol his wife had decided to try to tear his scrotum literally to shreds, and she had partly succeeded. She must have had very sharp nails . . . Six months after this incident they were divorced – the wound healed very nicely, though.

Men themselves also do weird things. When in the spring of 2006 Wales inflicted a painful defeat on England at rugby, 31-year-old Geoffrey Huish cut off his own testicles. He carried out the operation in ten minutes with a blunt pair of pincers. He then threw the testicles into a plastic bag and set off proudly for the pub to show his mates that he had been as good as his word. Only when he reached the pub did the heavily bleeding Huish collapse. His drinking companions kept the testicles in a beer glass full of ice. But once he arrived at hospital it was clear that there was no hope for the Welshman: he would have to go through life without balls, and subsequently spent some months in a psychiatric institution.

Six months after this idiotic gesture Huish explained the facts. 'I said before the match to my friend Gethin that Wales didn't have a hope in hell of winning. It wasn't a bet, I just said I'd cut my balls off if we won. So after the match I kept my word. I went to work with the clippers. It took about ten minutes and I was in a lot of pain, but I just went on. The pincers were so blunt that it was a difficult job. There was a lot of blood, though I'd expected even more.' He concluded on a philosophical note: 'I think about what I've done every day, but I can't give any reason why I did it. I had a lot on my mind and felt a bit down. Well, I can forget kids now. I'd still like a family, though, so perhaps I'll adopt.'

Contrasting with this ludicrous and at the same time gruesome story is a beautiful poem by Richard Newman called 'The Silence of Men':

> A man I've never dreamed of before walks
> into my apartment and sits in the green chair
> where I do my writing. He carries
> in his left hand a large erect penis
> which he places silently on the floor.
> The phallus begins to waltz to music
> I cannot hear, its scrotum a skirt;
> its testicles, legs cut off at the knees.
>
> I want to know why this disfigured
> manhood has been brought to me. I look up,
> but my guest is gone. His organ, deflating
> in short spasms like an old man coughing,
> spreads itself in a pool of shallow blood.
> The silence between us is the silence of men.

In the urological literature there are regular reports of human bite wounds to the scrotum. Such bite wounds are quite frequently complicated by a bacterial infection, and that also applies to dog bites. Post-treatment research at Groningen University Medical Centre showed that virtually all patients who had reported to A & E with bite wounds in the crotch had been attacked by a pitbull terrier.

In the past conscripts were taught that a vicious kick in the crotch was the best way of taking out a potential enemy. Nowadays there are martial arts from the Far East that have turned dirty kicking into a fine art. Women doing a course in self-defence learn how to teach manners to an attacker. That sensation will be familiar to every man who has ever sat on the saddle of his bike too enthusiastically. It is no accident that footballers forming a wall to keep out their opponents' free kick hold their hands over their crotch.

Such injuries are a source of embarrassment. Injuries to the scrotum are common in hockey and kick-boxing. They are extremely painful because of the previously mentioned remnants of abdominal membrane in the scrotum, which make the pain nauseating. If the kick or ball is hard enough, the cover of the testicle, the *tunica albuginea*, can even rupture. If this is stitched as soon as possible, there is a 90 per cent chance that the testicle will be saved. If things are allowed to take their course, the chance is only 50 per cent. The operation is almost always performed under general anaesthetic, gas or injection; local anaesthetic is insufficient.

The testicle collector

Human craziness takes the oddest forms. Years ago I was approached by a female second-year medical student with the question 'whether I as a urologist could get hold of a human testicle for her?' She was so beautiful I was too flabbergasted to give the only correct response, namely: 'Are you out of your mind?' With a sophisticated grin she told me that her father saved testicles . . . Still under her spell, I replied that everything that urologists and other surgical specialists saw fit to remove from a human being was always sent to the pathologist, who had the last word, especially important if we were dealing with an unpleasant disease. Anyway, the pathologist always decides, though in very many cases when it is too late for the patient! Years later I came across the same beautiful student as a doctor – you guessed: as a trainee urologist! One day I decided to use her as an intermediary to see her father, the testicle collector, and his collection. I didn't dare go without her accompanying me, as I kept getting flashes of *The Silence of the Lambs*.

The man I met had a grey beard fringing his face and spoke with a slight Amsterdam accent. He lived opposite a cemetery, and told me that it was full, but that a new one had been built just outside the village. He had once studied mathematics and had gained his doctorate in medicine with a thesis on cranial measurements in growing children. He told his story.

It had all begun with two tiger testicles from a well-known wild animal refuge. One spring day in a café the decision had been taken: he was going to start a testicle collection, with tiger balls as the foundation. The two tiger testicles had been removed by a famous vet, and were now on display in a village to the north of Groningen, together with the testicles of, for example, bulls, monkeys, stallions, hippopotami, sea lions, polar bears, cocks, camels, walruses, panthers, guinea pigs, llamas, tomcats, rats, water voles, and others too numerous to mention.

Only after long and persistent questioning did it emerge that there was a kind of testicle mafia behind his operations: doctors attached to well-known zoos, local pig castrators, vets from surrounding villages, a farmer from the village itself, a chicken keeper who still knew how to make capons, a globetrotter who went off to Egypt to castrate camels, *and* his enchanting daughter.

In the presence of his future son-in-law the testicle collector, who in my eyes was becoming increasingly reminiscent of Anthony Hopkins, informed me that he wasn't ruling out the possibility that at least one testicle of his future son-in-law would find its way into the collection. After a glass of wine I hastily beat a retreat.

Once she started training as a urologist the testicle collector's daughter also turned out to be slightly mentally disturbed: together with a young, friendly, red-haired fellow trainee she had the nerve to clean a dog's penis she had been given by a friendly vet – that is to remove all the flesh with a spanking new operating set in a sterile operating theatre, leaving nothing but the penis bone, which was what she was after. The whole mess cost a fortune, since the instruments could never now be used for operations on human beings. To my great surprise she was allowed to continue training as a urologist. Probably her fairly gullible red-haired colleague had taken all the blame on herself.

Punishments, wars, tortures

'He that is wounded in the stones, or hath his privy parts cut off, shall not enter into the congregation of the Lord', said Moses in Deuteronomy 23:1.

For the unsuspecting Bible reader this probably seems a very severe utterance. I couldn't make head or tail of it until I found P. Dufour F. Helbing's *The History of Sexual Mores in All Peoples and at All Periods*. And what happened at the time of Moses? Jewish men were in the habit of grabbing each other's genitals when fighting in order to win. Even their spouses joined in. In Deuteronomy 25 we read:

> When men strive together one with another, and the wife of the one draweth near for to deliver her husband out of the hand of him that smiteth him, and putteth forth her hand, and taketh him by the secrets:
> Then thou shalt cut off her hand, thine eye shall not pity her.

In order to put an end to the above-mentioned practices, Moses ordained that those who had been castrated or had their penis cut off would no longer be permitted to attended the congregation of Jehovah.

Bullet and grenade wounds to the penis belong more to our age. In the Vietnam War, in pre-Nelson Mandela South Africa and in recent years in Bosnia these have been documented extensively, as has castration. The latter humiliating procedure is as old as the hills. In the Middle Ages in particular men were castrated as a punishment for sexual misdemeanours or miscalculations.

In the twelfth century the testicles of Pierre Abélard, the great theologian and philosopher, were cut off after his elopement with his beloved pupil Héloïse. Abélard deeply mourned the loss of his manhood and wrote extensively about it in his memoirs. As for Héloïse, she was sent intact to a convent, and later gained fame as the head of an establishment called Le Paraclet, founded by her former lover. The two of them eventually found the same resting place in the cemetery of Père Lachaise in Paris.

It is said that Rasputin's sizable testicles and penis are preserved in a specially made velvet box. This crazy Russian monk died an unenviable death: he was poisoned, shot, raped, castrated and finally drowned. However, no one seems to know what has happened to the box, any more than we know what has become of Napoleon's private parts!

In 1934 Professor Johannes Lange published a monograph on *The Consequences of Castration in Adults – Illustrated with Reference to War Experiences*. Adolf Hitler is not mentioned in the book, but it is known that he lost a testicle, probably at the Battle of the Somme in 1916. He became what I once heard an up-and-coming urologist describe as a 'single-stoner'. Hitler's case is not absolutely certain: it might of course have been an innate abnormality. During the Second World War the Allies made fun of the Führer in the song 'Hitler Has Only Got One Ball', which was later recorded by Bette Midler.

Torture involving the genitals is typical of 'dirty wars' and, more especially of dictatorships. In *The Feast of the Goat* Mario Vargas Llosa devotes page after page to it. From 1930 to 1961 the Dominican Republic was ruled by a dictatorship of the worst kind. A certain Rafael

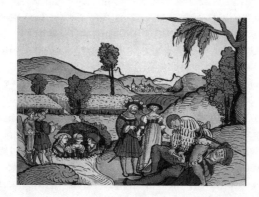

Castration of
the lover.

Leonidas Trujillo Molina ruled like a little Hitler. The writer gives an unvarnished and compelling picture of the absurd manipulations of this despot. After days of torture one of the rebels is slowly finished off:

> When they castrated him, the end was near. They did not cut off his testicles with a knife but used a pair of scissors, while he was on the Throne. He heard excited snickers and obscene remarks from individuals who were only voices and sharp odours of armpits and cheap tobacco. He did not give them the satisfaction of screaming. They stuffed his testicles into his mouth, and he swallowed them, hoping with all his might that this would hasten his death, something he never dreamed he could desire so much.

Chronic testicular pain

Men who have a tendency towards hypochondria quite often express this by complaining about their testicles. This may relate to a feeling of heaviness, a nagging or a stabbing pain. Complaints about such symptoms can become a source of frustration for everyone involved, the patient, the GP and the urologist. For the patient because he feels he isn't being taken very seriously, for the GP because he/she does not know what to do and for the urologist because by the time the patient is referred to him/her a great deal of frustration has built up and the urologist knows in advance that no objectively verifiable abnormalities will be found. So we are not talking about the acute pain of a twisted stalk of the testicle or the chronic pain of a swelling in the scrotum; with this pain a physical examination reveals no abnormalities.

Those affected are mostly relatively young, sexually active men, who have intermittent problems. Pain is signalled in one or both testicles, sometimes spreading to the groin. It is important to ask certain questions: when does the patient feel pain? Only during the day? Only when sitting for long periods or on the contrary when standing for long periods? Did the problem appear suddenly and continue from then on? Does the testicle pull towards the groin during an attack of pain? Does the pain sometimes pass when the patient is lying down? Has the patient undergone sterilization? Is there also pain during and/or after ejaculation? How frequent are the patient's ejaculations?

The physical examination of course comprises the careful feeling of the groin, the seminal cord, testicles and epididymides. The epididymis is normally sensitive to the touch, meaning that pain on contact by no means always points to an inflammation. Examination of the patient in a standing position is an absolute must (if medical students omit this in an examination, they fail outright). This can help one diagnose a rup-tured varicose vein as the cause of the nagging pain. In this case the person examining feels and sees a 'can of worms' next to the left testicle, which disappears when the patient lies flat.

When the patient is in a lying position the doctor can provoke the cremaster reflex by stroking the inside of the thigh or the lower abdomen. If the testicle pulls towards the groin and this is accompanied by the typical pain, the patient has an exaggerated cremaster reflex: because the muscle fibres are relatively too strong, the testicle is pulled into the groin. Information on this condition is vital; in extreme cases it may be decided to sever the muscle fibres in an operation.

Pain after a hernia operation can also occur and is caused by damage, which may or may not be temporary, to the tiny nerves that run along the inguinal canal to the scrotum. Generally speaking, patients often tell us that they only have a problem when sitting and when asked often turn out to have a sedentary occupation. Examples are taxi drivers, lorry drivers, sales reps, etc. In that case it is good to pay attention to clothing. Tight jeans are fatal to men with testicular pain – jeans are stiff and constrict the testicles.

Often testicular pain is related to sexual activities, since the patient sometimes has more pain during ejaculation or afterwards. It can some-times go on for days. It is not always clear whether this is connected with the degree of arousal, too much or too little sex. Think of Zorba the Greek, who one fine day, after a month of abstinence on an island where he has been doing some building work for an Englishman, says: 'I'm downing tools, I'm off back to the mainland – my groin is killing me.'

Often testicular pain is accompanied by pain in the area between the anus and the scrotum. This is usually wrongly diagnosed as chronic inflammation of the prostate when it is actually chronic pelvic pain caused by insufficient relaxation of the pelvic floor muscles. Treatment by a physiotherapist in such cases is often much more effective than long-term treatment with antibiotics.

Unfortunately there are by no means always ready-made solutions. Careful gathering of the facts is important, which in practice means taking the time to go through the symptoms and not giving the impression that one is not taking the case seriously. Chronic testicular pain is hard to treat. If the pain really derives from the scrotum and is not referred pain, severing the nerve pathways on a level with the external inguinal ring or a little higher will interrupt the conduction of pain sensation. If a trial blockage high in the seminal cord with a local anaesthetic results in a reduction in pain for the period for which the medication is presumed to work (for example, lidocaine one to two hours, marcaine three to seven hours), there are grounds for severing the nerves (denervation). A 'positive' blockage of the nerves in the seminal cord therefore also confirms that the pain actually derives from the scrotum. In addition the blockage has prognostic value for the success of the surgical denervation.

Epididyectomy, or the complete removal of the epididymis, *hemi-castration*, removal of the testicle *with* epididymis – and *vaso-vasostomy* (a restorative operation after sterilization) are also among procedures used to relieve patients' pain. Hemicastration is the most often recommended and most effective procedure. Quite tangentially, it should be mentioned that in the past hemicastration was used to determine the sex of the child to be fathered. If one wanted a boy the man's left testicle should be tied off. Left was associated with weak and right with strong. The Hottentots used the same method.

In hemicastration an approach through the groin is preferable because it produces better results than via the skin of the scrotum (leaving 76% of patients in comparison with 55% permanently pain-free). This difference may perhaps be explained by the high tying off of the seminal cord resulting in the complete severing of the genital branch of the nerve. Sometimes there are good reasons for completely ruling out surgical treatment; in such cases the patient is referred to the pain clinic for psychological treatment and/or medication.

Testicular cancer

. . . is rare: in the United States, between 8,400 diagnoses of testicular cancer are made each year. Over his lifetime, a man's risk of testicular cancer is roughly 1 in 250 (four tenths of one per cent, or 0.4 per cent). It is most common among males aged fifteen–40 years, particularly those in their mid-twenties. Testicular cancer has one of the highest cure rates of all cancers: in excess of 90 per cent; essentially 100 per cent if it has not metastasized. Even for the relatively few cases in which malignant cancer has spread widely, chemotherapy offers a cure rate of at least 85 per cent today.

Testicular cancer has several distinct features when compared with other cancers. Firstly, it has an unusual age-distribution, occurring most commonly in young and middle-aged men. Secondly, its incidence is rising, particularly in white Caucasian populations throughout the world, for reasons as yet unknown. And thirdly, testicular cancer is curable in the majority of cases. The number of deaths from testicular cancer in the USA is around 380 annually.

It is essential to discover the growth in good time. Very often testicular cancer causes few symptoms, at most a feeling of heaviness. Occasionally there is sudden pain because of a haemorrhage in the growth. One diagnostic trap is swellings that persist after a trauma or an inflammation of the epididymis.

In almost half of cases there is metastasis at the moment when a diagnosis is made. Possible symptoms are back pain, a swelling in the abdomen and breathlessness. Fortunately the prognosis is very favourable, even where there is metastasis. In most cases the metastases simply melt away with chemotherapy or radiotherapy. The choice between the supplementary treatments depends on the kind of cancer involved. Pathologists distinguish between *seminome* and *non-seminome*. In the first case the prospects are slightly more favourable than in the second.

The success stories of therapeutic chemotherapy in testicular cancer with metastases (for instance, Lance Armstrong) originate from cisplatinum. In 1966 the American biophysicist Barnett Rosenberg was playing around with a colony of intestinal bacteria, which he exposed to various levels of current between two platinum electrodes. The closer the bacteria came to the electrodes, the less able they were to divide. That was caused, thought Rosenberg, not by the electric current but by a substance on the platinum electrodes. That cell-inhibiting substance proved to be cisplatinum. When he went on to test the effectiveness of the substance on rats with cancer his intuition was confirmed. Further research showed that cisplatinum had an extraordinarily favourable effect on women with ovarian cancer and men with testicular cancer. When cisplatinum was first used on patients in the early 1970s it did, however, turn out to have a series of serious side-effects, including kidney damage, hearing loss and unbearable nausea. Nowadays those side-effects are successfully kept in check, for example by a combination of drugs, though long-term research indicates that premature heart problems may occur.

Besides cisplatinum, etoposide and bleomycine are used in the treatment of patients with testicular cancer. The number of courses is determined after a risk classification. During treatment so-called tumour-marker substances are identified in the blood, and in this way the success of the treatments can be assessed. In any case the side-effects of the chemotherapy remain severe: nausea, hair loss, reduction in bone marrow, anaemia, haemorrhages, pins and needles in feet and fingers, and lung damage.

Lance Armstrong

In 1992 Texan Lance Armstrong took the leap into the ranks of professional racing cyclists. A year later he became world champion road racing cyclist in Oslo. With stage victories in the Tour de France, etc. he emerged in no time as one of the best racing cyclists of his generation. In the autumn of 1996 this success story came to an abrupt end: Armstrong had testicular cancer with metastases. This was a bombshell – certainly in the world of cosseted racing cyclists, and his team lost a charismatic figure.

As Armstrong put it: 'My first reflex was: there goes my career. Later, when the seriousness of the disease sank in, I realized I'd be lucky if I was able to live a more or less normal life again. The doctors gave me a 50% of survival. The diagnosis was worrying to say the least: testicular cancer with metastases in the abdomen, lungs and brain.' The cyclist underwent two operations, in which, among other things, his right testicle and a brain tumour were removed. This was followed by three months of chemotherapy and intensive medical care in Indianapolis:

> For the first year not a day went by without my thinking about it, but since then the fear has begun to abate. I'm no longer just a cancer patient – I've become a racing cyclist again. I've got my ambition back. The will to win is back, although it's not as all-consuming as it used to be. I get over it quicker when it doesn't work out. Winning is no longer the most important thing in my life. I just enjoy each day as it comes. I kept cycling, even during that tough first year, purely for pleasure. When the doctors gave me the go-ahead, I decided to become a professional cyclist again. Eighteen months later I started my first race. Why? Because I love racing, because it's my job. But I also did it for everyone with cancer. Everyone thinks that after an illness like that you can never be the same again. I wanted to prove the opposite by winning races again. I'm gradually getting back to my old level. In fact, I've got even stronger.

Armstrong writes the way he cycles: straight down the line, always fighting openly and energetically. He's not the kind of man who hides. Even just after he had heard the bad news he did not avoid contact with the media. He fought the battle in the open. The Texan's openness won the respect of friends and enemies alike, in his team and elsewhere. And at a stroke testicular cancer became a topic in sports reporting and Armstrong became a representative of cancer patients.

His informal ambassadorship soon became official. In December 1996 he set up the Lance Armstrong Foundation, with the aim of fighting all forms of urological cancer by increasing awareness, education and research. Money is collected in the first place through all kinds of cycling events, the largest of which takes place each year at the end of May in his home town of Austin and is christened Ride for the Roses.

Bilateral cancer

Men who have once had testicular cancer are more at risk than 'normal' men of developing cancer in the remaining testicle. Synchronous bilateral cancer occurs in 0.7 per cent and 1.5 per cent develop cancer in the remaining testicle within a year. Only a small number of men are involved, but even so, imagine if it happens to you! Testicular prostheses and testosterone gel, though, make it possible to lead a normal life.

Generally speaking, as has been said, excellent treatment results are achieved with testicular cancer, certainly if one compares them with treatments of other types of cancer. Still the patients and all those involved are confronted with a totally different world. Information, mentoring and support are provided by patient support groups.

Testicular prosthetics

Testicular prostheses have been available since 1940. Before 1973 they were made of the metal vitallium, but since then gel-filled implants have been used worldwide. Prostheses are used, for example when:

- an undescended testicle has been removed
- a testicle has been removed because of a tumour
- a testicle has been removed because of a torsio testis that has been discovered too late
- where a testicle has been missing from birth

Why use a prosthesis? Many men feel incomplete without a testicle. Young men often use one because they do not yet have a sexual relationship, or are frightened of someone seeing, for instance, in the shower after sports or in the sauna or on the beach.

Testicular prostheses come in various sizes, and inserting one is a simple procedure: an incision is made just above the scrotum through which the prosthesis is introduced and if necessary attached. The operation takes about twenty minutes, so that the patient can return home the same day. Research has shown that complications occur only in exceptional cases, and these take the form of: leakage, mostly after a trauma, a haemorrhage, infection, wound dehiscence or an allergic reaction. In order to prevent infection the patient is given antibiotics before and after the operation. In most cases a prosthesis can be claimed on insurance.

In 1999 the radiographer Luca Incrocci from Rotterdam carried out a research project among men with a testicular prosthesis. He examined thirty men aged between eighteen and 75 who had a prosthesis implanted. The average age of the research sample was 30. With five of these men there were complications. A few results from this research: 20 per cent still had problems with sexual contacts, 20 per cent still had sexual problems, but almost 70 per cent experienced an improvement in body image after insertion of the prosthesis. The latter fact is significant, since that is what a prosthesis implantation is ultimately about! The other problems can in the great majority of cases be solved not through an operation but by consulting a sexologist.

Modern testicular transplantation

As mentioned in a previous chapter, at the beginning of the twentieth century testicular transplants were widely used with the aim of combating the ageing process. At the time there was absolutely no knowledge of the factors determining the ageing process and loss of potency. Attention turned to the testicles: testicular tissue, either human or animal in origin, was transplanted, mostly in sections, into the scrotum. Remarkable results were reported for a broad spectrum of ailments, though the research results were rather coloured by personal motives. The ensuing polemics damaged the development of endocrinology, the science of hormones. That was even more the case with the commercial exploitation of this irrational treatment. In 1935 testosterone was isolated, so that testicular transplants fell temporarily out of fashion.

Due to new technical capabilities in the surgical field new interest was awakened in testicular transplants in the 1960s. Experiments focused on rats and dogs and eventually led to the transplantation of an individual's own material, in particular with baby boys who had extreme forms of undescended testicles. Transplantation from one human being to another was initially carried out only in the then virtually inaccessible Soviet Union; virtually nothing reached the outside world. In the 1970s a publication appeared on a successful testicular transplant in a pair of monozygotic twins, one of whom had no testicles and the other two. Inspired by this, two Chinese research teams began a test transplant in human beings. Despite the limitations due to the suppression of rejection in the recipient, remarkably good results were achieved, and a report appeared on the first two children fathered with a transplanted testicle. In the view of the researchers testicular transplantation could be of crucial importance for, for instance, *anorchid* men (literally without testicles), a condition affecting one in 20,000 men. Anorchidy is not life-threatening but if untreated it leads to a loss of libido, psychological problems, premature ageing symptoms and accelerated loss of bone mass. A select group of men with fertility problems might also benefit from testicular transplantation. It could be used for couples who choose the possibility of having a child independently over new techniques of reproduction and for whom the disadvantages are outweighed by the above-mentioned advantages. Of course female-to-male transsexuals would be eligible for testicle transplantation, though as yet no transplantations from one man to another have yet been carried out. Quite apart from the ethical aspects, it is the side-effects of the medication required after surgery which are the main obstacle to the procedure.

chapter seven

Ailments of the Penis

You can always rely on a friend, so they say, and hence many healthy young men never stop to think that an erection isn't a natural occurrence for everyone. In medical jargon we refer to erectile dysfunction – ED for short: in fact, the word 'impotence' is no longer used. Typical erection problems occur when the penis does not become (sufficiently) erect, or when an erection does not last long enough for satisfying sex. Descriptions like 'not hard enough', 'not long enough' and 'satisfying' are of course highly subjective.

Many men have occasionally have found that their erection is not always equally strong, or sometimes even fails to materialize. 'Problems' requiring treatment arise only when symptoms persist for a longer period. ED can adversely affect one's experience of sex, can damage one's sense of self-worth and put pressure on a relationship. Many men experience not achieving an erection as a sign of inadequacy. As a result an erection problem can play into the hands of one's fear of failure, creating a vicious circle. Sometimes there is also embarrassment about seeking help, since it is estimated that only 15 per cent of men with ED consult a doctor. There are conflicting reports from researchers about the frequency with which erection problems occur. At any rate they are much more widespread than most people think.

It is clear that as one gets older the chance of ED increases. One's sexual appetite may flag somewhat with age, arousal is no longer so intense, the blood vessels are no longer so supple, other physical ailments appear and older men often take medication that adversely affects their erection.

Psychological or physical?

Not only patients but doctors too consider it important to decide whether the erection problem is caused by psychological or physical factors. Why is that? In the case of a patient with a duodenal ulcer not much attention is usually given to underlying psychosocial problems. A prescription for medication to inhibit or neutralize stomach acid is soon written out, and constitutes what is known as symptomatic treatment. In the case of ED, however, the patient does not get off so lightly: the experts must, as far as they can, determine whether the problem is psychological or physical in origin. That is probably why many men are ashamed to reveal their erection problems. Research by GPs showed that over 85 per cent of men with an erection problem needed help, but only 10–15 per cent had actually sought help. Once he has gone to his GP the man with ED who does not react, or does not react positively to an erection pill prefers to be referred to a urologist rather than to a sexologist. The former works with various types of apparatus, syringes and needles, or may decide on an operation. For many men that is obviously less threatening than having to talk to a sexologist about all kinds of details of their failed love life. Men have a relatively strong tendency to rationalize. Research into GPs' treatment methods showed that a consultation in which the erection problem is first broached lasts on average thirteen minutes, and in only 10 per cent of cases is the partner present.

The patient can, in the best-case scenario, expect the following questions: is the problem in getting an erection or in maintaining it? If an erection can be achieved, the blood supply is probably adequate. How long does the erection last? Does the erection disappear before or during coitus, and how long has the problem been going on? Is it affected by the position of the body? (In terms of coital position men are vulnerable in the missionary position: the moment they start making coital movements relatively more blood is channelled away towards their legs, which can be at the expense of the blood supply to the penis – certainly if there is hardening of the arteries. In a nutshell: 'It's a choice between sex and legs.' Other questions probing the cause of the erectile dysfunction include: are there any apparently unrelated physical ailments? What about the use of medication, alcohol, tobacco and drugs? Urologists also often use a questionnaire.

What is the situation among non-Western men? Is ED more common among them? Do they deal with the problem differently? According to GPs, Muslim men often broach sexual problems via a physical complaint. An erection problem may be presented as pain in the penis, knee or abdomen. The complaint is probably expressed in a veiled way because discussing psychosocial and sexual problems with an outsider is taboo in Islamic culture, while 'being ill' is accepted. Turks and Moroccans also generally expect to be prescribed drugs. Injections are more highly valued than tablets, powders or suppositories. With Turkish men potency and fertility are crucial for their sense of self-worth, vitality and pride. Consequently erection problems can be seen as a loss of vitality or even as the approach of death.

Psychosocial aspects of the problem are dealt with at length: is the ED linked to a particular partner (how do you ask that clearly and yet discreetly?), or is it connected with tiredness? Was there any unpleasant psychosocial event associated with the first occurrence of the problem? What are conditions like at work and what are the prospects, or are there perhaps worries that subconsciously demand too much attention? Has something happened to the permanent partner to make her/him less attractive? Are there nocturnal and morning erections and are you able to masturbate as before? How is your appetite for sex? What does the man actually think about the situation and how is his partner reacting?

In the first volume of his *Essais* the great French philosopher Michel de Montaigne (1533–1592) went into these problems at length. Montaigne wrote in a fluid, improvised style, with a string of associative leaps. He tells of a friend of his who had heard a man say that he lost his erection the moment he wanted to penetrate a woman. He was so overcome with shame at his flaccid member that the next time he was in bed with a woman he couldn't put it out of his head, and the fear that the same disaster would befall him again was so great that it prevented his member from becoming erect. From that moment on he was unable to achieve an erection, however much he desired a woman. The shameful memory of each setback tormented and dominated him more and more.

Montaigne's friend had become impotent when he lost his unshakeable rational control over his penis, which in his eyes was an essential component of normal masculinity. According to the philosopher Alain de Botton, Montaigne did not blame the penis: 'Except for genuine impotence, never again are you incapable if you are capable of doing it once.' Because of the frightening idea that we have complete mental control over our bodies, and the terror of deviating from the normal pattern, the man could no longer perform. The solution was to adjust the pattern, and render the event less traumatic by accepting that the loss of power of the penis was an innocent blip in one's love life. Montaigne took the unforeseen caprices of the penis out of the dark recesses of unspoken shame.

Montaigne knew a nobleman from Gascony who could not maintain his erection with a woman, who fled home, cut off his penis and sent it to the lady in question 'to make amends for his insult'. Montaigne had better advice:

Married folk have time at their disposal: if they are not ready they should not try to rush things . . . It is better . . . to wait for an opportune moment . . . Before possessing his wife, a man who suffers a rejection should make gentle assays and over-tures with various little sallies; he should not stubbornly persist in proving himself inadequate once and for all.

Examination of patients with erection problems

In the physical examination we check whether there is a normal pattern of male hair growth, we listen with the aid of a stethoscope to see if there are any indications of vascular constriction, and if necessary we test reflexes, and feel the penis and the scrotum.

Physical examination of a man with ED does not generally provide any information that was not already perfectly obvious. Nevertheless there are plenty of men who believe that their complaint is the first symptom of a serious disease, and unfortunately this is occasionally the case. In young men the danger is multiple sclerosis and in older men serious cardiovascular disorders. Other diseases which are known to cause erection problems are long-term high blood pressure, leukaemia, serious kidney diseases, hyper- or hypothyroidism, diabetes, underde-veloped or bilaterally damaged testicles, hyper- or hypoactivity of the hypophysis, overactive adrenal glands, amytrophic sclerosis (also an ailment of the spine), spinal cord lesion, serious epilepsy, hernia of the back, Parkinson's disease and, last but not least, inflammation of the prostate.

If cancer requires the removal of the prostate, bladder, or rectum, this also leads in most cases to ED. Because the surgeon has to keep a margin of healthy tissue around the tumour in order to ensure a last-ing recovery by the patient, it is inevitable that some nerves involved in erection will be damaged. It is hence extremely important that the patient should be informed of this before the operation. Radiotherapy can also cause ED.

Additional examinations

Under normal circumstances every man has nocturnal erections, the duration and hardness of which are related to age. Usually a man has such erections between three and five times a night for between twenty and thirty minutes as part of dreaming. In ED with a physical cause, nocturnal erections occur scarcely if at all. The first quantitative data on erectile capacity were obtained a few decades ago from test subjects' sleeping for a number of nights with a so-called erectiometer around the penis. These meters were nothing more than a felt strip with graduated markings. The following morning it was possible to check whether there had been nocturnal erections and if so how strong. The test was also carried out with the perforated edge around a sheet of stamps. If the following morning the border was found to be torn, this was more or less conclusive evidence of a nocturnal erection. Nowadays university hospitals have very sophisticated equipment for registering nocturnal erections, and thus determining whether an erectile problem has a psychological basis.

The blood supply and drainage can be assessed with the aid of duplex scanning. In this context duplex means simply that two examinations, namely echography and Doppler, are combined. The duplex measurement is carried out both at rest and after an intrapenile injection with a vasodilatory substance. This measurement is important in checking whether the ED is caused by arteriosclerosis. Using the echograph the arteries in the penis can be located, after which the flow can be measured with the aid of the Doppler sound signal. There is a light-hearted limerick on the Doppler effect:

> There was an old German named Brecht
> Whose penis was seldom erect.
> When his wife heard him humming
> She knew he was coming –
> An example of Doppler effect!

Only a minority of men with ED look for the cause in the psychological field. Mourning is often suggested, especially by widowers who after a while enter into a new relationship. A similar problem of course affects widows and divorced women, who also have to wait and see whether things click sexually. The snag is that the new partners – probably wrongly – expect to share the same bed as soon as possible, and under those circumstances a widower feels under pressure to prove his potency. The man has cared for years for a wife with failing health and after she dies he falls into an emotional black hole, and naturally the same would apply to a widow. Sadly, starting a new sexual relationship is by no means always easy for bereaved partners.

When it finally comes to sexual intercourse even young men may fail to come up to the mark, as illustrated in the following limerick:

There was a young fellow named Bliss
Whose sex life was strangely amiss,
For even with Venus
His recalcitrant penis
Could never do better than t

h

i

s

.

In most cases ED at a young age is an expression of shyness, though occasionally there is a serious underlying psychological problem.

ED can also be indirectly caused by young women: some are easily distracted, become bored when the experience turns out to be less exciting than they thought, or feel a mounting sense of rebellion. In such cases their deprecatory and sometimes insulting remarks can cause their young lover's penis to go limp. This happens especially if the man involved feels he has to give a terrific performance, while feeling extremely unsure of himself. Sometimes he is frightened of hurting his partner, and occasionally he imagines the hymen as a sort of drumskin, dense and stretched taut, which has to be perforated, causing excruciating pain when coitus is first performed.

Apart from that there are quite frequently anxieties regarding one's own sexual organ. One of the most common expressions of this is so-called *pseudophimosis*. The sufferer has never been taught how to observe proper penile hygiene, including thorough cleaning of the glans, so that with a strong erection and even more when entering the narrow vagina, he experiences a slight pain and a great deal of anxiety. The result is an abrupt termination of this first sexual approach and a disinclination to take any further initiatives. If a patient does not spontaneously raise the subject, but simply states that though he achieves a good erection, his organ becomes flaccid the moment the penis is introduced into the vagina, there are good grounds for a physical examination. If the man is asked to roll back his foreskin, he appears to try very hard but still does not manage to do so. If one tries to help him, one's offer is rejected. After some persuasion and with some trepidation he allows the doctor to expose the glans. At this point the person involved is quite frequently close to fainting. A large quantity of smegma shows that the foreskin has not been properly cleaned. Afterwards the man is urged to roll back the foreskin daily and wash his member with soap and water. This is the quickest way to overcome his fear of the vulnerability of his exposed glans. After this he will no longer find it difficult to entrust his precious organ to his partner.

Experience shows that resentment at adultery by the female partner can also become a malignant growth that eats away at potency.
Adultery itself also quite frequently leads to ED. The Italian feminist
Pia Fontana writes about an impotent adulterer in the story 'The
Diary', in which she describes how the protagonist, Elsa, seduces the
married cardiologist Riccardo. They had met at the house of friends,
after which she made an appointment at his surgery, not because of an
ailment, but with something else in mind. This only becomes clear to
Riccardo at their second meeting. Elsa is able to bring him to a pitch
of excitement, while at the same time realizing that making love surrounded by the usual metal cabinet full of files, a wrinkled cloth screen,
a treatment table covered with a strip of white paper and the inevitable
photo of wife and two children, is bound to be a terrible experience.
Elsa goes exploring and discovers a blue tiled bathroom. That's where
it will have to be, she thinks, turning on the hot tap:

> He caressed her, licked her, lay on top of her, and then some-
> thing embarrassing happened – embarrassing for him, that is,
> since Elsa didn't find it all that strange: despite everything Ric-
> cardo couldn't get it up. Well, it's nothing exceptional, but it
> was a nuisance, for both of them . . . He tried, tried again, but
> he just couldn't do it. And he was really in the mood, perhaps
> *too much* in the mood, or perhaps there was something else.

Elsa becomes irritated by his failure, while Riccardo repeatedly apolo-
gizes and maintains that he is completely under her spell:

> 'Why do you keep on trying?' said Elsa. 'It's really not that
> important to me, you know.' She dried herself with strips of
> paper – from the treatment table – there was a whole roll in the
> cupboard.

Riccardo can't stop apologizing, and as Elsa leaves the practice, she
reflects that he is a nice, interesting man. She smiles at the thought of
his failed attempts, but the two of them never have a second chance.

Divorce, tensions at work and suppressed homosexuality are also
well-known causes of ED. It is estimated that in America between 2 and
4 million people are married to a homosexual or bisexual partner –
usually without knowing it. Between 20 and 30 per cent of gay men
and women go into heterosexual marriages despite being aware of their
own sexual proclivities: 95 per cent of married homosexuals were
aware of their sexual preferences before marriage and 90 per cent had
had homosexual experiences. Most believed that marriage would 'cure'

them. According to an article in the *New York Times*, 15 per cent of American married couples in which one partner comes out as homosexual, remain married.

An illustration from my own practice: a well-groomed 53-year-old man attends the surgery for erection problems. His physical condition is good, though he suffers from diabetes and has to inject himself with insulin twice a day. Diabetes suggests a physical cause for his complaint, but not every ailment suffered by a diabetic patient is necessarily caused by diabetes. The patient has been married for nineteen years, by his own testimony happily. After a number of tests have been carried out it gradually becomes clear that his problem is not so much one of erection as of arousal. The man has nurtured homosexual feelings for years, but does not want to act them out. However, he wouldn't dream of divorce. He lives in a rather remote little village, and by his testimony coming out openly would be absolutely impossible. The patient feels very negative about referral to a psychologist-sexologist. The suggestion of establishing secret homosexual relationships in town is also dismissed out of hand. He does, though, make it clear that he would like to continue to be monitored every three months. The background to this wish only becomes clear when I have talked things through with an experienced female sexologist in a peer group discussion. She explains that for the man in question visiting a male urologist may count as a kind of sexual contact, which at least offers him the opportunity to speak frankly and openly about his feelings.

It is known that in the course of history some political leaders had potency problems while involved in a power struggle, particularly if the outcome was still uncertain. Mao Zedong was a well-known example. 'When his power climbed to great heights in the early 1960s, he seldom complained of impotence,' wrote his personal physician in a biography of the Great Helmsman. From an early age Mao was determined to remain healthy as he grew older and to remain sexually active until he was 80. However, pride came before a fall, and his personal physician was ordered to give him regular injections of an extract of ground deer antlers, which traditional Chinese medicine considers a potency-enhancing substance. There is no evidence as to whether the injections helped.

Like Mao, the majority of men with erection problems believe they have a physical ailment. The lack of an erection is equated with being ill. In the first instance therefore people want to be examined, and their organ is presented for cure or repair, preferably with pills or injections, or if necessary through an operation by the urologist, traditionally the plumber among doctors. Today the crux of the matter is increasingly: 'What's wrong with my body, and can the fault be repaired?' It's very rare for a man unable to get an erection to say: 'Stands to reason, I don't really feel like it.'

In the 1980s the previously mentioned psychologist Bernie Zilbergeld was considered one of the authorities on male sexuality. In his books he gives a compelling sketch of the still current image of the erect penis: 'It's two feet long, hard as steel, and can go all night.' To support that assertion he quotes extensively from popular literature, for example from *The Betsy* (1971) by Harold Robbins, one of the world's best-selling authors:

> Gently her fingers opened his union suit and he sprang out at her like an angry lion from its cage. Carefully she peeled back his foreskin, exposing his red and angry glans, and took him in both hands, one behind the other as if she were grasping a baseball bat. She stared at it in wonder.
> *C'est formidable. Un vrai canon.*

Partly because of these overblown images many men shrink to anxious bullocks whose members refuse to behave every day like a cross between a baseball bat, a raging lion and a cannon.

Occasionally someone is prepared to admit that his potency problem is connected with his partner: she bores him, there's no curiosity, no mystery any more, the excitement has gone. Getting into a sexual rut becomes the cause of ED. In this area it is obviously not only the vagina that has the right to strike – the penis does too. Sexologists call this the 'Coolidge phenomenon', after the American president Calvin Coolidge, who features in the following anecdote:

> One day the president and his first lady visit a state farm. Soon their guided tour splits in two. At the chicken run Mrs Coolidge asks the farmer how often a rooster mates. 'Scores of times a day, ma'am,' replies the farmer. 'Be sure to tell the president that,' says Mrs Coolidge. When the president comes along and is told about the rooster, his question is: 'With the same chicken every day?' 'Oh no, Mr President, with a different one every time.' Coolidge nods and says: 'Be sure to tell my wife that!'

Exclusive sexual relations with the same partner can be an advantage. In 1994 the psychologist W. Zeegers published *The Sunny Side of Sex: The After-Effects of Satisfying Sexuality*. In the book he compares the sex lives of couples, whom he divides into three categories: couples who always do the same thing in bed, couples who try to make each session of lovemaking something special and couples who invite others to share sex. They were selected on the basis of their own assessment that they enjoyed a satisfying love life. It was scarcely surprising that the various couples experienced sexuality differently: the way in which their experiences differed turned out to be much more interesting. With people who had a sex life with little variation things always went well: the partners never felt that any particular session was exceptional. It was naturally inconceivable for them that it might ever go less well. They never fantasized during lovemaking. Within this group there was clearly both love and intimacy, and apart from that each partner knew that the other would never do anything odd – it was just all very familiar.

Cultural influences

Our views on impotence are completely bound up with the time and culture we live in. The ancient Chinese, for instance, never saw the phenomenon of impotence as a significant problem. When the penis no longer became hard enough, the method of 'soft' entry was recommended, as described by Jolan Chang in *The Tao of Love and Sex*. If a man is experienced and dextrous enough, according to this old Chinese method, he can manoeuvre even a completely limp penis inside a woman. According to the Tao one must not attempt penetration when the vagina is not moist. If necessary, vegetable oil can be used as a lubricant. The key to the success of this soft penetration method is the man's dexterity. As soon as the penis has been manoeuvred into the vagina, he must make a ring round the base of the penis with his fingers with the aim of keeping the tip as stiff as possible. You might conclude that soft entry is a sensible technique for men with erection problems, but that a potent man will have no need of it. According to the Chinese tradition, however, this is definitely not true. 'Soft entry is not just for the beginner or the problem case. It is an integral part of the Tao of Love,' writes Jolan Chang. However, there is a snake in the grass. Soft entry and deferred ejaculation in fact serve only male self-interest. Men who want to live to a great age must according to the prescripts of the Tao replenish their weakening yang, the male essence, which is the source of strength, energy and a long life – with *yin shui*, the water of yin, or the vaginal secretions of young women. Because yang is essential for the health and energy of the man, he must not harm it. This is why a Taoist seldom ejaculates during coitus. Instead he tries to keep his strength up with the secretions of his female partners. The more yin shui he absorbs, the more the essence of the man is strengthened, which is partly why there must be very regular intercourse!

Similarly in the ancient Hindu culture, from approximately 4000 to 1000 BC, the solution to erection problems was sought not so much in the man himself as outside him, for example in eating a mixture of sesame seed, salt, pepper, brown sugar, eggs and buttermilk. The Hindus had many remedies for impotence, which were written down in the *Ayur Vedas*, meaning literally: 'Poems on the Knowledge of Life'. The best-known of these is the 'Sushruta Samhita'. In the Indian sex manual *Kama Sutra*, written in AD 400, great attention is given to the dimensions of the sex organ. On the basis of penis size men are divided into hares, bulls and stallions, while women can be hinds, mares or elephants. The *Kama Sutra* argues that the combination of a hare-man and a hind-woman leads to better sex than the combination of either of these two with a larger animal. Anyone wishing to follow this advice, though, encounters a practical problem: how many partners do you need to experiment with before you find the right size? In ancient India weak erections or overshort penises were also tackled with an ointment made of equal parts of myrrh, arsenic, aniseed and boric acid, mixed with sesame oil.

When, many centuries later, Frederick of Prussia lay on his deathbed debilitated by disease, his personal physician prescribed the company of a young woman. However, this was not a matter of potency. The doctor assumed that the spirit of a young person could pass into an older person, causing a kind of rebirth. At the time this phenomenon was called *sunamitism* after the Sunamite maid of King David in the Bible.

It is said of the legendary first emperor of China, the Yellow Emperor, the patriarch of the race of Han, from whom all Chinese are supposed to be descended, that he became immortal by going to bed with a thousand young virgins. The emperors who succeeded him all believed that the more sexual partners they had the longer they would live: hence their thousands of concubines. The first emperor of the Qin dynasty, Qin Shihuuangdi is said to have sent a Taoist priest and five hundred virgins across the sea in search of the elixir of immortality. According to legend the Japanese are the descendants of this priest and the five hundred virgins on the mission.

Nowadays the view is that the invigorating effect of young people on the elderly is mainly psychological in nature. Sometimes a young woman feels attracted to an older partner, sexually as well as in other ways. That can reach the point where it could be seen as pathological: a condition that until recently psychologists described as 'gerontophilia'.

Impotence in the Middle Ages

In the Middle Ages witches were often accused of having caused impotence. They could do this, for instance, by putting a spell on the member so that it disappeared completely into the abdomen; German witches especially were regarded as very skilled at this. The first person to link impotence and witchcraft was Hincmar, the archbishop of Rheims, who lived the ninth century. One of his pronouncements was that a man was not allowed to remarry after a divorce on the grounds of proven impotence from physical causes. However, if the impotence was the result of witchcraft, the victim was free to enter into a new marriage.

In addition witches were also charged with having sexual intercourse with the devil. The snag with this was that the devil's penis differed from that of a normal man. Some witches said that it was divided into two at the tip, forked and lithe as the tongue of a snake. This enabled it to be inserted both vaginally and anally, very like the method used by gynaecologists to examine their patients. The devil's member was remarkable in several respects. Stories circulated about how his penis was scaly and covered in barbs. Descriptions of the length of the member differed: from that of a little finger to that of an arm. Besides the shape, the composition of the organ was described as abnormal: it was icy cold, as hard as stone, half horn and half iron.

It goes without saying that vaginal contact with such an organ was not much fun! The prince of darkness's copulations, it was assumed, produced ever more little witches and caused his power to grow accordingly. In the Middle Ages there were hordes of incubi and whore devils, demons who in the shape of a man or a woman crept into someone's bed and copulated with monks and virgins, servants and mistresses.

The publication of *Der Hexenkammer* (The Witches' Chamber) in Cologne in 1487 is generally regarded as the beginning of the witch hunts, though in fact persecution had begun much earlier. This book, written by two notorious inquisitors, includes the story of a man whose penis had been whisked away by witchcraft, a case that today would be considered as an illustration of passing psychological impotence. Briefly summarized, the story is this: after ending his affair with a girl a young man promptly loses his member. His body has become completely smooth in the place it once occupied. He subsequently meets a woman in an inn who asks why he is so terribly sad. Her advice is to make the girl in question give him back his member, if necessary by force. He follows the advice and asks the girl to lift the spell.

When she pleads her innocence, he almost strangles her and says: 'If you don't give me back my member, I'll kill you.' The girl proves intelligent enough to play along. She puts her hand between his thighs and says: 'Here it is again,' From that moment on the young man has his penis visibly and tangibly back in place. The psychological origin of this impotence is clear, though the inquisitors interpret it in their own way: the penis has not been torn from the body, but has been magicked away by the devil!

In *De Praestigiis Daemonum* (1563) the Dutchman Johannes Weyer (also known as Wier) was one of the first to criticize the witch hunts. Impotence was also dealt with: Weyer demonstrated that this generally had a natural cause, for example the eating of certain herbs. In the event of impotence, he believed, one should not therefore base oneself on spells or accuse innocent people. Weyer did not deny that the devil can damage a man's reproductive capacity, but argued emphatically that Satan did not require any old women for that purpose. Weyer had no time either for miraculous cures for impotence. On hearing of a man who regained his potency after rubbing himself with raven's gall, Weyer's wise conclusion was that superstition can obviously not only harm but also benefit a man.

One can admire the psychological insight of this individual, who was able to put an end to the madness, not by saying that the devil was a fiction, but by taking him seriously and hammering home the message that with his lies about witchcraft he had played a nasty trick on mankind. In Weyer's view it was not the women indicted for witchcraft who were under the devil's spell, but their accusers: a sublime turning of the tables, which saved the lives of countless women. Weyer's name lives on in, for example, the Johannes Wier Foundation, a Dutch organization of obstetricians, doctors and nurses who oppose the violation of human rights and in particular defend the interests of asylum seekers.

While studying a fifteenth-century document found in Montpellier in France the medical historian Sigerist found an interesting treatise on impotence. It includes the statement that there are people incapable of coitus by reason of enchantment by the devil. If this befalls a man, he should address himself to God, who will grant him mercy. However, because there are different forms of spells, the writer of the manuscript feels obliged to deal with them all separately. Some spells are cast with the aid of animal substances, such as cock's testicles. If these are placed under the marital bed together with the blood of the cock, sexual intercourse becomes impossible. Another method is to cut a nut or an acorn in two and place it along the way to be taken by the married couple after the wedding. Another kind of charm is to hide letters written in bat's blood, and raw beans are also used, being most effective if they are placed on the roof or above the doorway.

Should the bride or bridegroom be the victim of one of the above-mentioned charms, it is better to talk about it than to remain silent, since those afflicted are disgracing not only themselves but also their relatives and are sinning against the Holy Ghost.

A few freely translated remedies:

A spell by means of letters can be recognized from the fact that the bride and bridegroom are not affectionate with each other. One must search both above and below the doorway, and if one finds anything one must take it straight to the bishop or the priest. If a nut or acorn is the cause, the woman must divide a nut or acorn in two, after which the man and woman, each holding one part in their hand, must stand opposite each other on the road, then walk towards each other and put the two pieces back together for at least seven days. After that they will again be able to have intercourse. In the case of a spell involving bones, this can only be lifted with the help of God.

The gall of a male dog cleanses the house and prevents it from being afflicted by any spell. If the walls are sprinkled with the blood of the dog the spells will also be annulled. If the bride and bridegroom collect fish gall and carry it in a basket made from the branches of a juniper bush and scatter it on the hearth in the evening, the spells will also be banished.

If the above measures did not work, the couple should consult a priest. After making confession the couple had the opportunity to take Holy Communion on Ascension Day. After partaking of the body and blood of Christ, the married couple were supposed to give each other the 'kiss of peace'. They were then blessed and sent forth with the urgent advice to refrain from any attempt at intercourse for three days and three nights, after which success was guaranteed! Centuries later the celebrated sexologists William Masters and Virginia Johnson were to incorporate the latter exercise in their therapy.

One may note in passing that doctors or would-be doctors are not exactly famed for their fantastic sexual prowess. They have plenty of excuses: busy, irregular working hours, the great emotional demands made by their work, and so on.

Back to the Middle Ages: Nicolas Famel (1330–1418), a celebrated scholar at the University of Paris, was both an exorcist and an alchemist. He believed that rotting wood was extremely effective with impotence-related problems, but it must be first soaked for three days in the urine of a sixteen-year-old virgin.

One of his other remedies was as follows:

Take some burdock seed; place it in a bowl; mix it with the left testicle of a three-year-old billy-goat, a pinch of powder made from hair from the back of a completely white dog which you have cut on the first day of the new moon and burnt on the seventh day. Pour all this into a bottle half filled with brandy; leave this uncorked for twenty days, so that the stars can do their work.

On the twenty-first day exactly, the first day of the next new moon, boil everything until the mixture thickens to a paste; then add four drops of crocodile seed and strain the mixture through a cloth.

After collecting the liquid in a bowl, you need only rub the parts of the impotent man with it, and he will perform wonders. This mixture is so effective that there have been cases where women have become pregnant simply through the intimate rubbing of the man.

Since crocodiles are quite rare in Europe and since obtaining the seed of this animal is extremely difficult, it may be replaced with the seed of various kinds of dog. Apparently that is possible because dogs are so strangely agile in eluding the eager jaws of a crocodile. On the banks of the Nile these dogs are very common. In any case, we are assured, the above experiment has been repeated several times and up to now it has always succeeded, with both dog and crocodile seed.

Medication

In the last century it was also believed that certain medicines could adversely affect potency. Roubaud described how in the treatment of tuberculosis with iodine vapour he saw four cases of impotence develop. Saltpetre also acquired a bad reputation. The use of bromide compounds mainly affected sexual desire. Camphor dulled the sensitivity of the genitalia.

Today it is mainly medication for lowering blood pressure and psychoactive drugs that have a bad name. The same applies to a number of drugs to counter arrhythmia, Parkinson's disease, certain medication prescribed for excessive stomach acid production and drugs used in treating prostate cancer. Some of the drugs mentioned adversely affect the desire for sex, others impede the stiffening of the erectile tissue compartments in the penis or lead to a 'dry' climax, meaning that sperm is forced into the bladder. Doctors call this phenomenon retrograde ejaculation. It is always worthwhile discussing with the prescribing doctor whether alternative medication is available.

Within the medical profession itself there is an ongoing debate about whether it is or is not advisable to point out possible unwelcome side-effects to patients before medication treatment starts, especially with side-effects of a sexual nature. It is desirable to ask about the patient's sex life before starting treatment, so that the patient knows that the doctor is prepared to discuss the subject. Apart from that, it is a way of establishing whether or not the man has problems in this area. If it is necessary later to check whether there is a possible connection between sexual problems and the drug, this information can be useful.

On the other hand it is not fanciful to suggest that even the mention of, for instance, possible erection problems when using medication to counter high blood pressure, may become a self-fulfilling prophecy. These days, however, patients read the package inserts and ask questions on their own initiative about possible side-effects. In such a case the doctor will point out that these phenomena are quite rare, and it is impossible to predict who will suffer from them. As has been said, in the event of side-effects it is sensible to confer.

Yet it still happens that patients make a connection between their sexual problems and the drugs they are taking, but do not dare to raise the subject. They may even discontinue taking the medication without telling their doctor. Because, say, their blood pressure is not dropping sufficiently, they are prescribed a higher dosage or more medication, which they still do not take, and so on . . . Asking about sexual side-effects now and again in check-ups can provide an opening for a full discussion, and will undoubtedly benefit the patient's adherence to the treatment.

Alcohol and drugs

Quite a few men believe that a steady intake of alcohol heightens potency – but this couldn't be further from the truth. Chronic excessive alcohol consumption can lead to all kinds of sexual problems. Alcohol attacks the body in various ways: in the long run both the central and the peripheral nervous system can be affected. The substance also has a toxic effect on the testicles. Besides that less testosterone is produced and the liver is progressively less able to break down oestrogen (men also produce a small amount of this female hormone).

In the nineteenth century the effect of various kinds of wine was a serious object of study. The German physician V. G. Vecki believed that the heavier dark-red wines like Bordeaux, Dalmatian and Californian wines and some Spanish varieties have a positive effect on potency.

Champagne was in his view pernicious, increasing the libido but harming the erectile apparatus.

The porter's famous description of the effects of alcohol in *Macbeth* still rings true: 'It provokes the desire, but it takes away the performance.' Shakespeare's point is still valid: excessive drinking is bad for the erection mechanism. It is sometimes said of impotence that it is a matter of wanting but not being able. In the case of excessive alcohol consumption, however, the reverse usually applies: one is able, but doesn't want to.

Nicotine reduces potency through its vascular constrictive effect, meaning simply that the blood supply to the penis is reduced. Research with dogs, which were required to inhale a fixed quantity of nicotine, proved this beyond question. The effect of recreational drugs depends partly on the way in which they are used (smoking, snorting or intravenous injection) and the level of the dose. In addition, it is not exceptional for several drugs to be used simultaneously. Marijuana, methadone and heroin not only lower the testosterone level in the blood, but also result in a raised prolactin level. An excess of that hormone (which triggers milk production in nursing mothers) reduces the desire for sex.

Too high a prolactin level in the blood is fortunately only very rarely the result of a *prolactinoma*, a tumour affecting the hypophysis. Depending on its size it must be treated by medication, radiotherapy or operation.

Congenital abnormalities

Some years ago there was a discussion about whether someone born with a serious disorder of the external sex organ could have a satisfactory sex life as an adult. When a survey was conducted among adult men with an 'open' bladder (*exstrofia vesicae*) and the accompanying seriously abnormal (short) penis, it was found that seven of the eleven were satisfied with the way they functioned sexually, though the other four were clearly not. There is very little research of this kind to be found in the scientific literature.

In his posthumously published diaries, *The Business of Living*, the Italian writer Cesare Pavese (1908–1950) describes his own life as a lost battle. Pavese was impotent because of a congenital defect in his sex organ. He talks of a struggle with his own character, which over the years he came to regard as an insurmountable fate. When Pavese put an end to his life in 1950, it was the culmination of something he had been heading towards for years. There has been much conjecture and much has been written about why he committed suicide: criticism and misunderstanding from the Communists, the fact that no woman was prepared to commit herself to him, but mainly his sexual problems.

A few fragments from the diaries:

7 December 1937: A man who has not come up against the barrier of some physical impossibility that affects his whole life (impotence, dyspepsia, asthma, imprisonment, etc.) does not know what suffering is. In fact, such causes bring him to a decision of renunciation: a despairing attempt to make a virtue out of what is, any case, inevitable. Could anything be more contemptible?

23 December 1937: The child who passes his days and nights among men and women, knowing vaguely but not believing that this is reality, troubled, in short, that sex should exist at all, does he not foreshadow the man who spends his time among men and women, knowing, believing this is the only reality, suffering atrociously from his own mutilation? This feeling that my heart is being torn out and plunged into the depths, this giddiness that rends my breast and shatters me, is something I did not experience even when I was befooled in April.

The fate reserved for me (like the rat, my boy!) was to let the scar heal over, and then (with a breath, a caress, a sigh) to have it torn open again and a new infection added.

Neither deception nor jealousy have ever given me this *vertigo of the blood*. It took impotence, the conviction that no woman ever finds pleasure with me, or ever would. We are as we are; hence this anguish. If nothing else, I can suffer without feeling ashamed: my pangs are no longer those of love. But this, in very truth, is pain that destroys all energy: if one is not really a man, if one must mix with women without being able to think of possessing them, how can one sustain one's spirits and vital power? Could a suicide be better justified?

25 December 1937: If screwing was not the most important thing in life, Genesis would not have started with it.

Naturally everybody says to you 'What does it matter? That's not the only thing. Life is full of variety. A man can be good for something else,' but no one, not even the men, will look at you unless you radiate that power. And the women will say to you: 'What does it matter,' and so on, but they marry someone else. And to marry means building a whole life, a thing you will never do. Which shows you have remained a child too long.

Spinal cord lesion

A spinal cord lesion is a catastrophic event. There is an abundance of therapies for this group of mostly young patients: physiotherapy, water therapy, psychotherapy, you name it. But sex therapy is not on the list. Not only many professional helpers, but family members and others believe the patient will never again have a sex life. The unspoken question they are asking themselves is to what extent someone can love such a badly injured body.

The writer D. H. Lawrence (1885–1930) takes this as his theme in his once shocking but now classic novel *Lady Chatterley's Lover* (1928). The main character's husband is a war invalid, who at the age of 29 suffered a complete spinal cord lesion. His wife is six years younger. It so happens that the husband, Clifford, proved emotionally cold even before his injury. With great artistry Lawrence describes Lady Chatterley's passionate relationships: first with Michaelis, whose 'pathetic two-second spasms' cannot ultimately satisfy her, and later with Mellors, the gamekeeper, the embodiment of the natural male element and the complete antithesis to her wheelchair-bound husband.

Particularly in the initial post-traumatic phase many spinal cord lesion patients see sex as a closed chapter, something that is no longer compatible with their badly damaged body image. At a later stage spasticity or stiff joints may hamper sexual activity, and there may also be involuntary loss of urine during sex, especially if the bladder is not emptied in advance. One positive aspect is that new erogenous zones may develop, such as nipples, neck, earlobes or the skin in the transitional area between those parts of the body with and without sensation. Sexual need is particularly great among these patients without a partner. That need is catered for, for example, by the TLC Trust (www.tlc-trust.org.uk), which provides counselling and sexual services, and by discussion forums for the disabled like that at www.thesite.org.

A new technique, still in its infancy, is a neurological bypass. This involves an operation to redirect a nerve from the groin to the head of the penis, which requires the damage to the spinal cord to be below the point where the inguinal nerve branches off from the spinal cord, that is, below the first lumbar vertebra. The operation was first performed in the Netherlands with spina bifida patients. It often takes at least six months before any kind of sensation returns and it may take two years before it is possible to assess how pleasant that sensation is. The brain has to learn that signals are no longer coming from the groin, since at the beginning a touch to the glans is registered in the groin. The man himself has to begin to (re)associate the sensation in the penis with sex.

If there is a partner and she is responsible for most of the care, that may be to the detriment of the sense of their being lovers. Friction between partners, one of whom is handicapped, often relates to that care. 'If you have a row with your wife and half an hour later you have to ask her to put you on the toilet, it's no joke,' as one spinal cord lesion patient told me. Experts advise that the seriously handicapped are best cared for by a professional rather than by the partner, which is a way of preventing the carer–patient relationship from coming to replace love and friendship.

Partners wanting to end a relationship with a spinal cord lesion patient may feel a certain guilt, which can lead to the postponement of that decision. This may stem from a feeling of responsibility and concern about what will become of the invalid partner. It is important to distinguish love and pity: in the view of some psychologists staying with someone out of pity is a mistake. Others believe that love can develop into empathy: the sense of experiencing and sharing the other's suffering. That does not detract from the fact that it can be a very hard decision, especially if those around one take the side of the person left behind. Lady Chatterley chose to leave after she become pregnant with Mellor's child and her husband refused a divorce – and who can blame her?

Wedding-night impotence

One day I was rung up by a psychologist to ask if I would teach a patient to inject himself in the penis. The case was as follows: a young Turkish man was due to leave for his homeland to collect his wife. They had only been married for a few weeks, but unfortunately his bride had been taken back home because the poor bridegroom had been unable to achieve an erection on their wedding night. His wife remained a virgin, bringing shame on her family. On the principle of 'now or never', the unfortunate man was taught how to inject himself: if things didn't work spontaneously, he would have some chemical backup. He left with needles, syringes and a number of ampules of vasodilatory fluid. A few weeks later we heard that fortunately everything worked without injections, and that the patient had been able to display the bloody sheet proudly to the family.

In the story 'Le moyen de Roger' (Roger's Method) French writer Guy de Maupassant (1850–1893) paints a very accurate psychological picture of an initially disastrous wedding night. A young Parisian couple, Roger and Gabrielle (who is a widow), plan to celebrate their wedding night quietly at the bridegroom's apartment. Consumed by passion and desire, they soon withdraw to the bedroom, but Roger, the brand new bridegroom, finds it impossible to achieve an erection:

When I joined her in bed, I lacked confidence in myself, I admit it. I felt edgy, troubled, ill at ease.

I took my place beside her as a husband. She said nothing. She looked at me with a smile playing round her lips, visibly anxious to make fun of me. This ironic attitude, at such a moment, finally disconcerted me and, I admit, robbed my arms and legs of their strength.

When Gabrielle realized my . . . embarrassment, she did nothing to reassure me, quite the contrary. She asked me, in an offhand way:

'Are you as full of life as this every day?'

I couldn't stop myself answering:

'Do you know you're insufferable?'

Then she started laughing again, but laughing in a quite immoderate, unseemly, exasperating way.

It's true I cut a sorry figure, and must have looked very silly.

From time to time, between two paroxysms of hilarity, she said, choking on her words.

'Come on – that's the spirit – put some energy into it – my – poor darling.'

Then she broke into such helpless laughter that she couldn't stop giggling.

Rage and humiliation drive the young husband into the street. In despair he determines to put his manhood to the test, follows a prostitute to her room, and lo and behold, succeeds with no problem in doing what he had failed to do half an hour before. With a restored feeling of self-worth he returns to the hotel where he acquaints his wife, herself a-tremble with trepidation and excitement, with the delights of love, this time with an erect penis.

In Japan wedding-night impotence is still a frequent occurrence, presumably prompted by the very different sexual mores of the country. Wedding night impotence undoubtedly occurs in other countries too, but often for quite different reasons: many bridegrooms overindulge on the big day, or even more often, are too tired.

Adultery

Almost two thousand years ago the Apostle Paul's pronouncement that it is better to marry than to burn in hell was a reluctant admission that human sexuality must have some sort of outlet. Marriage – the institution within which sexuality was to be experienced – was thus accepted by the church – though not yet blessed: that came only later. This view of St Paul's had far-reaching consequences for Western civilization.

The story of Anna Karenina, told by Leo Tolstoy (1828–1910) and set in Czarist Russia, is deeply sad. Trapped in a marriage with Karenin, twenty years her senior, Anna travels with her family to St Petersburg, where she meets Count Vronsky. Vronsky is a professional soldier, a gifted horseman and a man of honour, and does what he can to avert the impending disaster. But their feelings cannot be suppressed, they fall hopelessly in love and – as is common in an extra-marital relationship – become increasingly reckless and careless. When the affair reaches Karenin's ears and he publicly disowns his wife, Anna's status and life are shattered, and she finally throws herself under a train. Vronsky suffers no more than a setback to his career.

People will go on being unfaithful until the end of time. Playing away retains its attraction, even for people who in practice never indulge. The fact is that many people are unfaithful in their fantasy: 60 per cent of women and 80 per cent of men fantasize about sex with someone other than their own partner. Figures on actual adultery differ so widely that it is difficult to say anything conclusive about them. It probably happens more frequently than we think. However, we are left with the problem that ED quite frequently occurs with adultery, since the man often feels guilty about deceiving his partner. Guilt sometimes also derives from the awareness that one is being unfeeling and cruel to the person one is deceiving. Many men realize that they can no longer truly love their partner, and the same probably applies to women: adultery causes one's partner, male or female, great suffering and painful humiliation.

A poem by Johann Wolfgang von Goethe (1749–1832) illustrates this point. In 'The Diary' he describes meeting a pretty young woman at a country inn. There is an immediate spark of attraction, and very soon they find themselves in bed, but at the crucial moment his penis leaves him in the lurch. The poet describes the accompanying feelings of rage and shame: 'My master player, hitherto so hot,/Shrinks, novice-like, its ardour quite forgot.' He is a prey to anxiety and despair. 'Better a bloody foe/In battle than this shame!' 'I raged a thousandfold, my soul was rent/With cursing and self-mockery both at once.' He cannot comprehend why he cannot perform better. Then the mood of the poem changes. Despite his failure, his bedfellow is satisfied, having experienced love and tenderness:

> How chaste she was! For though she made me free
> Of her sweet body, loving words, a kiss

Contented her; she nestled close to me,
Desiring, as it seemed, no more than this;
Happy she looked, peacefully, yieldingly
Satisfied, as if nothing were amiss.

The real moral of Goethe's poem is that male impotence is a divine punishment for adultery. Wasn't the sacrament of marriage after all instituted to combat promiscuity and ensure that the reproduction of the species took place in an orderly manner? Imagine the general surprise at an article that appeared in a newspaper on 18 April 1995 under the headline: 'Bishop: adultery in the genes.' In the article Richard Holloway, Anglican bishop of Edinburgh, was reported as saying that the church should not condemn adultery. 'Man can't be blamed for being unfaithful. It's how God made him. It's in the genes,' said the bishop. This statement was part of a series of lectures in which he wanted to take sex out of the taboo sphere. The response of the head of the Anglican Church, despite the appeal to genes in mitigation, was unambiguous: 'Adultery is and will remain a sin.'

The bishop probably has a valid point. Human beings are not innately monogamous: the vast majority of cultures recorded by anthropologists are polygamous. Sociobiology sees men as having a deeply rooted urge to supply their sperm to as many women as possible, just as women prefer to receive as many suppliers as possible in order to optimize the chance of pregnancy. That would explain why so many people – both men and women – have such a problem with monogamy: the spirit is willing, but the flesh is weak. That is definitely not just a matter of our Judaeo-Christian cultural roots. Who cannot feel Othello's genuine jealousy? He loves Desdemona and his jealousy is mingled with the fury of the insulted husband. This kind of jealousy – clearly timeless – should not be confused with the feeling of besmirched honour.

The only possible answer to the question of the jealous husband, of Othello: 'What are you thinking, what are you feeling?' is the pathological answer of masochism, self-torment. Where adultery has been proved, the only way out is love itself: surrender, acceptance of the freedom of the loved one. Impossible? Perhaps, but it is the only exit if we are imprisoned by jealousy. Love can exist only by the grace of freedom. In the view of the Mexican writer Octavio Paz freedom in love is a great mystery, a paradox that grows in a psychic substratum which unfortunately also contains poisonous plants like faithlessness, betrayal, jealousy and forgetfulness.

An unsatisfactory partner

Some men are unable to find real satisfaction with their own wives, though they have no problem at all with other women. The problem is partner-linked, and there is a host of possible reasons. For almost three decades Bernhard Premsela (1890–1944) worked as a GP in Amsterdam. In addition he was medical director of the Aletta Jacobs Family Planning Institute. Over the years he had heard every possible question about sexual matters and learned how to answer them – including questions about partner-linked impotence. He did many people a service by recording his experiences in *Sexology in Practice* (1940). However, in the chapter describing the psychological causes of 'relative impotence' in men, it is women who come in for severe criticism:

> A slovenly appearance is often responsible. Some women believe that once they are married there is no further need to take care about clothes or toilet. They look sloppy; a neglected face and hands complete the picture. Don't misunderstand me: I'm not arguing for rouge, lipstick and plucked eyebrows. I deplore this kind of make-up, which turns the average woman into a herd animal and robs her face of all personal cachet – which is precisely what gives it its charm. I mean only that pleasant grooming, which keeps the women and marital relations fresh and fascinating. Any woman who neglects such things, may pay dearly for this failure, with her husband's relative impotence.

A little later he has this to say about odours:

> For many partners alcohol-drenched breath is an insurmountable obstacle to achieving an erection. I believe this phenomenon is more common that is usually believed. Some people find tobacco smells from the mouth or on the fingers a powerful arousal-dampening factor, though I have also known cases where the smell of a cigar or pipe, but especially of cigarettes, had exactly the opposite effect.

On excessive hair growth:

> There are women who even when young exhibit a different pattern of hair growth from the average. Two aspects may have an inhibiting effect on the man's libido. Firstly, body hair. The average woman has only armpit hair and pubic hair, the upper

limit of which – as a secondary sexual characteristic – is marked by a horizontal line. Many women diverge from this norm and have a more or less virile pattern of hair growth (no horizontal upper limit to the pubic hair, but a diamond-shape, ending at the navel; hair-growth on breasts, arms and legs).

I saw many cases where impotence had resulted from excessive hair on the thighs, sternum or breasts. The second aspect, which can have a powerful inhibiting effect on the emotions, is hair growth on the upper lip and chin. This may vary from a very light down above the lip, which some men find very attractive, particularly in dark-skinned women, to the forming of a moustache or beard. The latter may extinguish all sexual feelings. The cure is the removal, preferably as soon as possible, of the *corpora delicti*.

Of course Premsela's points are overstated, but some of them may ring true. At the same time one needs to realize that 'clothes maketh the man' is not an empty phrase. Many women find sexual relations with their beer-bellied spouse a far from pleasant experience!

In fiction too partner-linked impotence is a much-discussed topic as, for example, in Milan Kundera's *Farewell Waltz*:

> 'I'm really tired,' he said.
>   She took him in her arms and then led him to the bed.
>   'You'll see how I'm going to make you forget your fatigue!'
>   And she began playing with his naked body.
>   He was stretched out as if on an operating table. He knew that all his wife's efforts would be useless. His body shrank into itself and no longer had the slightest power of expansion. Kamila ran her moist lips all over his body, and he knew that she wanted to make herself suffer and make him suffer, and he hated her.

'Professional' impotence

Some men are in love with their work, and put all their energy into it – which can lead to problems. One of these is described by the sexologist Wolfgang Buhl in *Eros mit grauen Schläfen* (1962): 'professional impotence'.

Buhl also speaks of 'scholarly impotence'. Any academics who feel under attack can console themselves with the thought that they are in good company. Louis XIV of France, Emperor Napoleon I, the composers Beethoven and Mahler, and the writers Gustave Flaubert, John

Ruskin and Bernard Shaw were known for their inadequate sexual performance. The impotence of many mathematicians and scientists is a matter of record: it is even said of Sir Isaac Newton that he never experienced full sex in his life.

Total concentration on work may gnaw away at erotic interest. Basically this is more a matter of not wanting than of not being able. This freely chosen way of life is no problem at all for workaholics. They themselves feel no deprivation, unless a conflict arises with their partner, who feels neglected, sexually as well as in other ways. Buhl illustrates with the example of Heinrich E., an engineer approaching 50. He has been married for twelve years to a wife ten years younger than him. A serious marital crisis leads the engineer to seek help. He tells his story: 'It's possible she sometimes finds me a bit odd, when I'm so absorbed in my work that I don't see or hear anything, but I always thought she'd got used to it. Of course she feels somehow excluded, but she just doesn't have a clue about technical things.'

The crisis turned out to have been triggered by a 40-year-old journalist, who Heinrich had got to know in the course of his work. Subsequently, 'because his wife wanted different people around for a change and not just colleagues of mine and their endless shop talk, he invited him to their house.

> He was an easy talker, whereas I don't usually say much. I think my wife knows perfectly well that there isn't much behind all those words – but, well, the guy was giving her something that I wasn't. I knew that nothing had happened yet, as they say, when I asked my wife what she really thought of the guy. She replied that I must have forgotten that I was a man and she was a woman. And she was right.

Then the tormented engineer describes his attempt to satisfy his wife sexually, which was a miserable failure. The therapist explains that it was not so much the long abstinence but the sudden pressure behind his resolution that was to blame for the fiasco:

> 'You still had one foot in your profession, so to speak. You must forget that as quickly as you forget this crisis. Just as you have to devote yourself completely to your work to make it succeed, so you must give yourself over completely to love. A long holiday with your wife is the best thing for you. Far away from it all, you have the best chance of regaining what you've forgotten,' said his therapist.

It is still true that some men are in love with their job, and in fact the practice ought to be banned in a collective wage agreement, though those involved wouldn't stand for that. Doctors too can work too hard or too much, disrupting their love lives.

Only a minority of men are able to use sex to recharge their batteries: however tired, they are always up for it (President John F. Kennedy was a case in point). That does not apply to most of us.

Wandering thoughts

What is your record sustained erection time in sexual intercourse? was the question put by Kinsey to several thousand American students. And what was the result? For 4 per cent it was under five minutes, for 18 per cent between about six minutes and a quarter of an hour, for 19 per cent between a quarter of an hour and half an hour, for 26 per cent between half an hour and an hour, for 14 per cent between one and two hours, for 5 per cent between two and three hours and for 4 per cent for three hours or more. Older readers will undoubtedly have to think hard, since you establish your record in your youth. Quite a few men lose their erection prematurely because they unconsciously assume the 'onlooker's role'. Their thoughts wander, they cease to participate in intercourse and their erection droops. In his *Confessions* (1781) Jean-Jacques Rousseau (1712–1778) describes such an experience, a failed adventure with the Venetian courtesan Giulietta, at length.

Full of passion, he appears at her bedside, but no sooner has he been able to see her in all her beauty than a thought arises in him that moves him to tears and completely distracts him from his original intention. He develops the thought more and more fully and his desire evaporates:

> Suddenly, instead of the fire that devoured me, I felt a deathly cold flow through my veins; my legs trembled; I sat down on the point of fainting, and wept like a child.
>
> Who could guess the cause of my tears, or the thoughts that went through my head at that moment? 'This thing which is at my disposal', I said to myself, 'is nature's masterpiece and love's. Its mind, its body, every part is perfect. She is not only charming and beautiful, but good also and generous. Great men and princes should be her slaves. Sceptres should lie at her feet.

The adventure eventually ends in a shameful fiasco. The young Jacques notices that the courtesan has a malformed nipple. He describes it at length and, inevitably, places the responsibility for his impotence at the door of the courtesan:

I beat my brow, looked harder, and made certain that this nipple did not match the other. Then I started wondering about the reason for this malformation. I was struck by the thought that it resulted from some remarkable imperfection of Nature and, after turning this idea over in my head, I saw as clear as daylight that instead of the most charming creature I could possibly imagine, I held in my arms some kind of monster, rejected by Nature, men, and love. I carried my stupidity so far as to speak to her about her malformed nipple. First she took the matter as a joke and said and did things in her skittish humour that were enough to make me die of love. But as I still felt some remnant of uneasiness, which I could not conceal from her, I finally saw her blush, adjust her clothes, and take her place at the window, without a word.

The scene ends with the now proverbial exclamation by the disappointed and angry courtesan: *Lascia le donne e studia la matematica!* (Give up women and study mathematics!)

Injuries to the penis

Erectile dysfunction may also be the result of a trauma to the penis. An unexpected movement during intercourse, unforced or otherwise, or during masturbation can cause a tear in the wall of the erectile tissue. The position in which the woman mounts the man back to front is the riskiest: the penis may bend in half against the woman's pubic bone. The tear is usually accompanied by a snapping sound, which is why urologists refer to it as a 'fracture of the penis'. An operation to stitch the tear is the only correct remedy.

A woman threatened with rape is therefore best advised to try to break her attacker's penis with her hand. Another option is to tense the pelvic floor so strongly that the man breaks his penis in his forced attempt at penetration. If a man presents with a fracture of the penis, a urologist with a sexological background will always keep the possibility of a sexual crime or at least rough sex at the back of his mind.

In the urological literature there are regular reports of human bite wounds to the penis. Oral sex has obviously still lost none of its popularity. These types of bite wound are quite frequently complicated by a bacterial infection, and there is also a risk of transfer of a hepatitis or HIV virus. One of the potentially unpleasant results of oral sex is described in John Irving's novel *The World According to Garp*, which evokes the life of a young writer in 1960s America.

Garp's wife Helen, in revenge for Garp's infidelity, has begun an affair with one of her students. While Garp is away at the cinema with the children, Helen tries to convince her lover, Michael, of her intention to end the affair. They are standing in the driveway of the Garp family home. Michael finally agrees to disappear from her life for good provided she gives him one last blow-job – in the car – as they have often fantasized about:

> He let one hand stray to the back of Helen's neck, which he gripped very tightly; his other hand opened his fly.
>
> 'Michael!' she said, sharply.
>
> 'You always said you wanted to,' he reminded her . . . 'But it wasn't safe, you said. Well, now it's safe. The car isn't even moving. There can't be any accidents now,' he said.
>
> Michael Milton had allowed her to see himself with what struck Helen as necessary vulgarity. *Suck him off*, she thought, putting him into her mouth, and *then* he'll leave.

She realizes that after ejaculation men usually quickly cease their demands, and her experiences in Michael's flat had taught her that in his case it wouldn't take too long. And time is of the essence. If Garp and the kids have gone to the shortest conceivable film, she has just twenty minutes. So she sets about it with determination, as if it were the last phase of a tiresome chore . . .

Garp and the kids return from the movies earlier than expected: the film turned out to be a dud. As usual, Garp drives the last stretch with the lights and engine off and turns into the driveway. But there is already a car in it . . . and the inevitable happens:

> Helen's head was flung forward, narrowly missing the steering column, which caught her at the back of her neck . . . Helen's mouth was snapped shut with such force that she broke two teeth and required two neat stitches in her tongue.
>
> At first she thought she had bitten her tongue off, because she could feel it swimming in her mouth, which was full of blood; but her head ached so severely that she didn't dare open her mouth, until she had to breathe, and she couldn't move her right arm. She spat out what she thought was her tongue into the palm of her left hand. It wasn't her tongue, of course. It was what amounted to three quarters of Michael Milton's penis.

Garp breaks his jaw in the crash and cannot speak for quite a while. In one of the notes he uses to communicate with his wife, he writes: 'Three quarters is not enough!'

Fortunately injuries to the penis cause generally only temporary problems. A well-known example is getting the penis caught in one's zip. In a hospital surgery department the zip problem is usually solved by removing the piece of foreskin that has caught in the zip with a knife, which has proved to be the least painful way. The zip has a double symbolic message, which can be summarized in two adjectives: 'mechanical' and 'sexual'. And it is the combination that makes it powerful: mechanical sexuality, but also injured sexuality. The zip is an instrument of seduction and an instrument by which the penis, erect or otherwise, can be injured.

Urologists are sometimes subject to great stress. A Romanian colleague of mine lost control when during an operation on a patient's testicles he accidentally severed the urethra. It was the last straw for the stressed-out doctor. He took a scalpel and, cursing, amputated the whole penis. While his female assistant looked on in astonishment, the surgeon placed the member in a tray and (chop! chop! chop!) sliced it up like an expert cook. Dr Naum Cioran is reported to have been fined 153,000 euros.

In the early 1970s there was a rash of non-medical penis amputations: in Thailand over a hundred abused women saw this as the only way of solving their problems. The penis was usually thrown out of the window, after which the ducks could gorge on it (the local houses were on piles, and ducks were kept underneath. Only in eight cases was reconstructive surgery carried out. In 1993 the whole of America was enthralled by the 'penis trial'. Lorena Bobbitt, a 23-year-old manicurist, was put on trial for cutting off her husband's penis. While drunk, he had repeatedly raped her – until she could take no more.

The proceedings turned into a parade of expert witnesses, doctors, psychologists and criminologists. There were hours of discussion on the significance of the penis as a power symbol. The case was regarded by a number of feminist groups mainly as a 'battle of the sexes'. Although her crime was not condoned, these groups maintained that any sentence would be a slap in the face for all women who had ever been abused. Lorena fortunately stayed out of prison – it was no coincidence that the feminists had threatened to castrate a hundred American men if she were put behind bars!

Nine months later – predictably – the video film *John Wayne Bobbitt . . . Uncut* was released. As part of the publicity campaign ex-nightclub worker Bobbitt made no secret of how wonderful it was to star in a porn video. When asked if it wasn't taking things a little far to use a porn film to show that his penis was working normally again, he replied that since everyone was curious anyway, he could convince them that he was in perfect working order. 'Despite the fact that sex still hurt a bit now and then,' said Bobbitt.

After Lorena, taking revenge on one's partner by cutting off his penis became quite popular: on average, one penis was amputated every two weeks.

I know of one literary story that shows some similarity with Lorena's. In 'Something Completely Different', Giuseppe Culicchia describes what a woman is capable of if she is treated with indifference by her husband. The woman is desperately unhappy, and cannot believe she was ever in love with her husband. Swearing and getting drunk is all he's now capable of. Moreover, he is pathologically jealous of his wife, whose career is flourishing; he is getting nowhere in his own job. One day the woman happens to go into an ironmonger's and sees an electric saw on display. On impulse she asks the salesman if the saw is really sharp, and when he says yes she decides to buy it, without yet really knowing what she intends to do with it.

One day her husband comes home drunk yet again and after a stream of verbal abuse, followed by rape, he falls asleep. Then she decides to use the saw:

> She unwound the long cord and plugged it in after unplugging the television. Then, very slowly, she pulled back the sheets. As usual Guido was sleeping peacefully. He always slept soundly. He had hairy legs. Barbara pressed the red button. The young guy in the shop was right. The electric saw cut like a knife through butter.

Women can also, as was shown by a newspaper report, cut their husband's penis off out of love. In 2006 Uta Schneider, a 65-year-old woman from Stuttgart, cut off the penis of her deceased husband. She wanted to preserve the sex organ as a souvenir of a very happy 35 years of marriage. She used a butcher's knife to relieve her dead husband Heinrich (68) of his member. She wrapped her booty in foil and was about to take it home in a lunchbox, when she was intercepted by a nurse and arrested for mutilation. 'It was the best part of him and gave me so much pleasure,' she said. 'I wanted to preserve it and keep it forever. We used to call it his "joystick" and I wanted that part as a memento,' she was quoted in *The Sun*.

War and torture

It is not only in war that gunshot wounds to the penis occur. Recently a fifteen-year-old boy was admitted to our hospital after being sprayed with buckshot by a pimp, and wounded in his private parts. How did this happen? Together with some boys of his own age he had got talking to a prostitute sitting at a window. Not only in her view, but also in that of her protector the conversation went on for too long. They didn't get down to business, so the youngsters were told to leave. They were foolish enough not to do as they were told, and the dramatic result was a blast of buckshot in the crotch. One of the eight bullets on target hit him in the middle of the right erectile-tissue compartment. After circumcision the skin of the penis was stripped off – the way one cleans an eel – and after much searching the piece of buckshot could be removed. Fortunately the urethra was undamaged.

During the Arab–Turkish conflict at the beginning of the twentieth century the Arabs had the gruesome habit of amputating the penises of Turkish soldiers killed in battle and stuffing them in the victims' mouths. The assumption was that if the dead man went to heaven, he would at least no longer be able to experience any sexual pleasure . . . More or less the same happened during the war in former Yugoslavia, when prisoners-of-war, it is said, were forced to eat the penises of their dead brothers-in-arms.

The ancient Egyptians practised penis amputation on a grand scale. In about 1300 BC the Egyptian commander Menephta returned from a campaign in what is now Lebanon, bringing with him 1,235 severed penises as war trophies! This deed is commemorated in hieroglyphics on a monument in Karnak. In the Bible (1 Samuel 18) we are told how Saul dispatches his son-in-law-to-be to fetch his bride-price: a hundred Philistine foreskins. In fact it was Saul's vengeful intention that David should perish in the attempt. However, David succeeds in securing not a hundred but two hundred foreskins, and Saul gives David the hand of his daughter Michal in marriage.

'Torture' by women has also been reported. In the chapter in which he explains why he firmly believes that the penis is considerably more sensitive than the vagina, the sexologist Havelock Ellis mentions a man who consulted him with a swollen, itchy penis:

> The wife, the night previous, on advice of friends, had injected pure carbolic acid into the vagina just previous to coitus. The husband, ignorant of the fact, experienced untoward burning and smarting during and after coitus, but thought little of it, and soon fell asleep. The next morning there were large blisters on the penis, but it was no longer painful.

At the time of the consultation the foreskin was retracted and puffy, the whole penis was swollen, and there were large raw patches on both sides of the glans.

Perverse thoughts

It is impossible to write about erection problems without dealing with the question of abnormal, deviant or perverse sexuality. The modern view is that a sexual act is not perverse provided it is performed by adults and that neither of the partners suffers any physical or mental harm. This makes it extremely difficult to establish criteria for what is supposedly normal and what is perverse. Take anal sex, for example. In the past Dutch farmers were wont to distinguish between their wives' weekday and Sunday holes (I'm afraid I've forgotten which orifice was associated with the Lord's Day).

Speaking of beastly thoughts: the Roman emperor Nero was subject to waves of incredibly capricious erotic fury. He often cloaked himself in animal skins, disguised now as a wolf, now as a lion, now as a swan, now as a bull. He would then attack chained prisoners, clawing them, biting them or mutilating them for his pleasure. In orgies he sometimes assumed the woman's role. He was convinced that no one was free of some kind of taint, and that no one was chaste, such are the apocryphal stories surrounding him. The wretched Nero died weeping in the arms of his wife Sporus. She was very careful that her blood did not mingle with that of her bestial husband, whose whole body was covered in stinking sores as a result of his endless sexual dissipation.

Whatever the case, sexual perversity is difficult to define, mainly because opinions differ according to time and place. In his wonderful book *The Inner Brothel*, Hans Plomp (1944) describes the adventures, as amusing as they are weird, of a perverse art critic. Though Plomp is not usually counted among the 'greats' of literature, for initiates he is a woman-friendly writer, which is greatly to his credit. In the book Barels the art critic becomes virtually impotent after a particularly unpleasant experience during intercourse. He has secretly turned the mirrors of his wife's dressing table in such a way that he will be able to observe himself during copulation. He hopes that she will fall asleep as usual during their lovemaking. That will give him plenty of time to play the voyeur . . .

One evening he is very insistent and though she isn't in the mood at all, she lets him have his way. As expected, she quickly falls asleep. Actually he quite likes that, as he can't stand her staring up at him while he is pumping away on top of her: she always has such an uninterested, disdainful expression. He carefully pulls the covers back. The sleeping woman gives a brief grunt when disturbed, but doesn't wake. Barels looks in the window behind him. There is only one lamp on the bedside table, but he can still see his pasty white buttocks reflected in the glass. He strains to get a better look, and suddenly he freezes. In the mirror he sees his wife's lower body, though lying on it is not himself, Barels, but a mangy grey-white dog with bare patches on its back and behind. The animal leers disgustingly at him. Barels catches his breath and lies absolutely still. Barels raises an arm, and a front paw is raised in perfect time. He breaks out in a sweat:

> He reaches for the light cord at the head of the bed and pulls on it. In the light he can see the animal quite clearly. It looks like a scurfy jackal. Barels groans in horror and to his astonishment it sounds like the growling of a dog. His wife is immediately wide awake. 'What are you lying there howling like a dog for? Please let me get some rest. I've got a headache and you're clammy with sweat.'
>
> 'Can't you see anything different about me?' asked Barels.
>
> She looked at him again with that disdain of hers. Then she said: 'You're a bit like a drowned dog, but that's nothing unusual.'

From that that night on Barels is virtually impotent. His few attempts turn into miserable failures. To make matters worse he has weak intestines, which gurgle dreadfully when he has just got into bed. Barels also confesses that he has found the cure for his impotence in the diaries of James Joyce, the Irish genius who knew no greater pleasure than lying under his wife's bottom so that she could relieve herself over him. Hadn't Joyce also written: 'The smallest things give me a wonderful hard-on – a brown stain on the back of your panties.' After Barels' confession his wife decides to leave.

Hans Plomp's story shows convincingly that every man is susceptible to perverse, bestial fantasies. What matters is what you do or don't do with them! Shouting them from the rooftops doesn't seem like a good idea – unless you want to make money out of them, of course.

Elvis Presley

On 28 October 1957 in the Pan Pacific Auditorium in Los Angeles Elvis Presley gave a legendary performance, his first in the city where he lived. A horde of stars with their children had turned up for the first of the two shows, in which Elvis shocked his audience with the steamiest, horniest antics most of them had ever seen. These involved an on-stage replica of Nipper, the famous mascot of the RCA record label. Elvis came on stage in the celebrated gold jacket and black wide-legged trousers, and for an hour gyrated his hips across the stage. But it was his last song that produced the headline: 'Elvis Presley will have to clean up his show – or go to jail.' No one knew what got into him, but when he launched into 'Hound Dog' his eyes had a wild look, and his pupils were dilated, as if he were very far away. He did the unthinkable: he began unbuttoning his trousers at the waist and pulling down the zip. The audience, already whipped into a frenzy by the sexual undertones of the show, went crazy.

With his trousers undone – though not dropped – Elvis grabbed hold of Nipper. He forced the animal against his crotch and started making masturbatory gestures. When the audience went completely wild, Elvis started rolling about on the floor with the replica of Nipper in a perfect imitation of bestiality. It was deeply shocking. The next day the vice squad arrived in suits with official warnings and a video camera. Elvis toned things down and Nipper's double came through the show unscathed.

Elvis would soon acquire the nickname of The King, but ironically the supposedly dangerous rock 'n' roll idol was anything but a sexual glutton. He wasn't that keen on intercourse, though he did like fellatio. This was connected with the fact that his mother had taught him that sex before marriage was a sin, and recalls Bill Clinton's proverbial protestation: 'I did not have sex with that woman!' Virtually impotent from medication and recreational drugs, Elvis departed this life on 16 August 1977, at the age of 42.

Solutions

Spanish fly, musk, garlic, grey amber (made from rotting whale intestine), vanilla, phosphorus, saffron, opium, chocolate, truffles, mushrooms, asparagus, strychnine, parsnips, ginger, cocoa, figs, calves' brains, shellfish, pickled meat, French beans, dried peas, red wine, marrowbone, fresh egg yolk, aromatic showers focused on the 'area', cold enemas, all kinds of mineral water, acupuncture, electropuncture, galvanic currents, electric friction, cauterization of the prostate, rest cures, milk straight from a nursing mother, are just a fraction of what has been recommended as a cure for potency problems.

Spanish fly is traditionally the best-known substance. It is made of the dried and powdered insects of the species *Lytta vesicatoria* from Southern and Central Europe and in Asia, which are about 2 cm long. The active ingredient is cantharidine, which when applied to the skin causes a powerful rash. Scientifically, the operation of the substance comprises both inhibition of phosphodiesterase and protein phosphatase activity and stimulation of beta receptors, causing vaso-congestion and inflammatory reactions. An oral dose of 5 mg gives a powerful stimulus to the urogenital system, but this dose can also cause severe kidney damage. Other side-effects include a burning sensation in the mouth, nausea, vomiting blood, blood in urine, epileptic fits and arrhythmia.

If Spanish fly has always been the best-known aphrodisiac, in the pre-Viagra period yohimbine was considered the best. At the end of 2006 the outgoing conservative-liberal Dutch government banned its use in herbal mixtures because of possible side-effects. Yohimbe bark comes from *Pausintyalia yohimbe*, a variety of tree from tropical West Africa. The South American quebracho tree (*Aspidosperma-quebrach-blanco*) also provides yohimbine. The substance inhibits the sympathetic nervous system. In high doses it is supposed to increase the blood supply to the sexual organs. If it is injected into the brains of rats, the number of copulations increases. Partly for this reason it is thought that yohimbine acts mainly on the brain. The scientists are agreed that yohimbine's possible effect is confined to psychogenic ED. The recommended dose is 10 mg daily, and possible side-effects are dramatic: heavy perspiration, giddiness, palpitations, falling blood pressure, overexcitement, trembling of the hands, insomnia, restlessness, hyperventilation, rashes, nausea and vomiting. An excellent move by an outgoing government!

In Greek mythology Aphrodite was the goddess of love and beauty, the daughter of Uranus, the personification of heaven. She has given her name to the term aphrodisiacs. Since the beginnings of recorded history man has been interested in aphrodisiacs, and in every culture people prepare love potions in the hope of restoring their potency or increasing it at will. The oldest description of an aphrodisiac is to be found in the Museum of Turkish and Islamic Arts in Istanbul, where a clay tablet from the thirteenth century BC contains the following (Hittite) cuneiform inscription:

> If the man's potency wanes in the month of Nisannu, you must catch a male partridge, pluck it, wring its neck and salt it; next mash it together with the Dadanu plant. Serve this mash in beer, after which you will soon see that potency is restored.
>
> You can do the same with the penis of a male partridge, the saliva of a bull with an erect penis or of a goat with an erection.
>
> Then take a sheep and make a ball of its tail hair and wool from the perineum. Tie this to the man's thigh bone and his potency will return.

Genesis (30:14–17) also contains references to an aphrodisiac:

And Reuben went in the days of the wheat harvest, and found mandrakes in the field, and brought them unto his mother Leah. Then Rachel said to Leah, Give me, I pray thee, some of thy son's mandrakes.

And she said unto her, Is it a small matter that thou hast taken my husband? And wouldest thou take away my son's mandrakes also? And Rachel said, Therefore he shall lie with thee to night for thy son's mandrakes.

And Jacob came out of the field in the evening, and Leah went to meet him, and said, Thou must come in unto me; for surely I have hired thee with my son's mandrakes. And he lay with her that night.

And God hearkened unto Leah, and she conceived, and bare Jacob the fifth son.

Mandrake is mentioned in one other place in the Old Testament, in The Song of Solomon 7:13: 'The mandrakes give a smell, and at our gates are all manner of pleasant fruits, new and old . . .' Mandrakes could be found while harvesting. They were extremely rare and were sought after not only for their wonderful scent, but because they were a cure for infertility. They contain mucous material, sugar, resin, non-volatile oil, tannin and various salts.

In Southern Europe it was believed for centuries that the mandrake grew mainly in places where criminals were hanged. According to tradition while in their death throes on the gallows they not only had an erection but also ejaculated. This sperm, consigned to the ground under extraordinary circumstances, was supposed to produce fertile ground for the mandrake. Christ's agony on the cross is almost never depicted with an erection. I am aware of only one exception: Maarten van Heemskerck's painting of Jesus that hangs in Ghent, which displays not only the stigmata of his crucifixion but also an erect penis. The association between strangulation and sexual excitement was later also a theme in the books of the Marquis de Sade.

The ancient Druids venerated the mistletoe, an evergreen, sticky, globe-shaped parasitic bush that lives on trees and never makes contact with Mother Earth, which they saw as a magic plant. The Gauls regarded it as a gift from the gods implanted in trees by lightning. They considered it a bad omen when parts of the plants fell out of the tree. The white-robed Druids cut the mistletoe at New Year ceremonies, probably the origin of the English custom of hanging mistletoe in the home at Christmas. The plant also had medicinal uses. Panoramix, the old, venerable druid from the village of Asterix and Obelix, would cut the mistletoe with his gold pruning knife to prepare the magic potion with which he made his people invincible. 'But he knows many other recipes . . .' says the writer, expressing the unspoken thoughts of the adult comic-book reader.

Things were different again with the Romans. Alongside the official physicians there were the so-called *sagae*, most elderly prostitutes. They operated in two areas: as unauthorized midwives who performed abortions or prepared magic potions with an aphrodisiac effect. Just like today abortions were carried out for a variety of reasons (other than because of a prenatally diagnosed harelip): a married woman, for instance, wanted to erase the traces of adultery, or a promiscuous woman was frightened of having her style cramped by lack of libido due to pregnancy. A few women took a different view: Julia, the daughter of the emperor Augustus, would only tolerate lovers when pregnant by her husband Agrippa. If people expressed astonishment that despite all her debauches her children always resembled her husband, then according to Macrobius she always said: 'I never take passengers, except when the ship is fully laden!' (*Etenim nunquam nisi navi plena tollo vectorem!*)

Though the abortions gave the *sagae* plenty to do, they still made up only a small proportion of their work. Normally these potion-makers came at night to the Esquiline Hill, which was the scene of magic spells and sacrifices, and the site of the cemetery for slaves, who were buried at random without even a shroud. It was unsafe there at night, and at the bottom of the hill close to the Porta Metia, stood the gallows and the crosses, from which hung the bodies of those executed. The executioner's house was naturally close by, since he had to watch over his victims. In these macabre surroundings the *sagae* did their work. By moonlight they picked their magic herbs and gathered hairs and bones and fat from those who had been hanged. According to Dufour there were even child sacrifices, particularly when very potent drinks had to be brewed. The *sagae* were paid handsomely for these dreadful practices. The child in question had first to be stolen from its wet nurse or parents, then buried alive and finally butchered. Otherwise the liver, the gall, the prepubescent testicles and the bone marrow would lack the true aphrodisiac power . . . Some *sagae* had the ability to produce potions that could make a man completely impotent, a fate that Romans dreaded.

The official, respectable physicians strongly disapproved of the use of all these potions, and countered by recommending natural mineral water rich in sulphur and iron, which must, though, be drunk close to the source. These *aquae amatrices*, as these invigorating drinks were called, lost their strength the further away from the spring they were drunk. So much for the Romans.

Since time immemorial musk has been considered an aphrodisiac scent. It is the secretion of the glands in a deer's foreskin, and the name derives from the Sanskrit word for testicle, an allusion to the fact that the substance comes from the sex organ. In nature musk smells are found in many places: the musk mole, the musk ox, the musk duck, the musk hyacinth, the musk cherry, musk wood, etc. In the mating season lizards and crocodiles secrete musk through glands in their lower jaw, and elephants do the same through glands in their head.

The mustard plaster was invented by Hammond, a nineteenth-century expert, who believed that this form of therapy must be used with caution, since it might cause inflammation or even cancer.

Occasionally there is a scientific explanation for the effect of a supposed aphrodisiac. In evolution it was the male boars who with their rooting and trampling spread truffles through a large part of France. Truffles are a type of fungus that grow underground among the roots of oaks and hazel trees. They are considered a delicacy and nowadays truffles are hunted with specially trained sows or bitches, the only creatures capable of detecting where the fungi are located. The clue to their ability is alpha-androsterone – a hormone – which makes these females wrongly think that they are on the track of a male. Since alpha-androsterone is also found in men's armpit sweat and women's urine, it is possible that it has an unconscious effect on sexuality.

The Chinese regard soup made from a sea swallow's nest as the ultimate aphrodisiac. The nest is made of sea grass held together with roe, a rejuvenating substance. In addition, sea grass contains a great deal of the previously mentioned phosphorus.

The Japanese walnut (*Ginkgo biloba*) is another medicinal source well known to the Chinese. The extract of the leaves is supposed to help the smooth muscle cells in the erectile tissue compartments relax and hence bring about an erection. The ginkgo has existed for hundreds of millions of years, originating in the Permian period, which means that herbivores like dinosaurs already grazed on ginkgo leaves in the Jurassic period. The tree is the only surviving intermediate form between the higher and lower plants, between the ferns and the conifers, though it is not a conifer but a deciduous tree. Fossil remains show that today's ginkgo has scarcely changed in the last 65 million years. A different, but scientifically interesting aspect, is that its swimming spermatozoids play a part in reproduction – an exceptionally rare occurrence in plants and trees. The ripe seed has a soft, fleshy yellow outer layer and the unpleasant smell of rancid butter. These seeds ('nuts') are prized as a delicacy in the Far East. The ginkgo disappeared from Europe in the Ice Age, and it was not until 1691 that the German doctor and botanist Engelbert Kämpfer, who worked for the Dutch

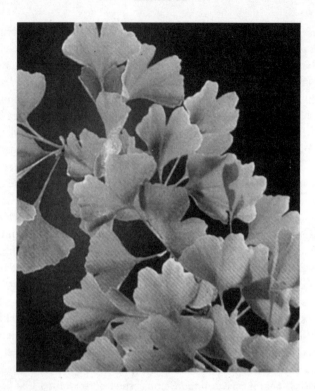

Gingko biloba leaves.

East India Company, rediscovered the tree in Japan. In the Far East ginkgos were regarded as very special trees, and in China had been planted from time immemorial in Buddhist temple and monastery gardens, where they were regarded as sacred.

In the temperate climate of Western Europe ginkgos grow quite slowly. The trees in say, Kew Gardens, are far older than most in Europe, but even they pale before the temple ginkgos of the Far East, some of them between two and three thousand years old, up to 20 metres in circumference and 60 metres high. The unique fan-shaped leaves, with a notch in the middle, turn a wonderful yellow colour in autumn. No wonder that Goethe devoted a fine poem to the tree. Ginkgos are no longer a rarity to be seen only in historical parks and botanic gardens: nowadays some can even be found lining suburban streets. The tree is indestructible, not even succumbing to an atom bomb. The death toll in Hiroshima was huge and massive buildings were completely destroyed, but the *Ginkgo biloba* only one kilometre from where the bomb landed simply went on growing.

Ginseng root comes from traditional Chinese medicine and is mainly used in Western phytotherapy to increase stamina. The major supplier is Pannax Ginseng from Korea. Its effect is supposedly based on an increased production of nitrogen oxide in the erectile tissue compartments in the penis. Nitrogen oxide is a potent vasodilatory molecule and the discoverers of that fact were awarded the Nobel Prize. With a little imagination one can see a little man in the shape of the ginseng root. So according to the doctrine of signatures, according to which the form and medical application of a plant are linked, ginseng is suitable for use with men.

In Asia the enduring interest in all kinds of aphrodisiacs has unfortunately resulted in the virtual extinction of both the Javanese and the Sumatran rhinoceros; the African rhino is also seriously under threat. It is widely believed, especially in East Asia and the Middle East, that the use of ground horn can restore potency, which may be associated with the fact that the act of mating in rhinoceroses takes almost an hour and involves multiple ejaculations. The horn commands astronomical prices and in Europe in the autumn of 1994 it reached the point where on the advice of Interpol rhinos in zoos were kept under close surveillance, since information had been received that poachers – a ruthless bunch anyway – were targeting animals in captivity.

Not so very long ago, on the island of Curaçao in the Netherlands Antilles, the iguana was in danger of extinction. Soup made from this splendid creature was supposed to eliminate potency problems. The iguana's sex organ is so shaped that it appears to have two penises, and a similar abnormal shape was once diagnosed in a human being, the 22-year-old Portuguese gypsy João Batista dos Santos. According to the doctors both penises functioned properly, and once he had climaxed with one he immediately continued with the other. The patient preferred the left-hand one, which was thicker.

There is a rice-based alcoholic drink in China that includes one lizard per bottle. This is a gecko (*Japaloua Polygonata*), a large species of Asian lizard, and the potent beverage is called Ha Kai Chiew. The Chinese attribute a salutary effect to the juices of the quick and agile gecko, especially in cases of impotence. The so-called 'preserving' of animals is traditional in many countries: in France adders disappear into eau de vie, in Spain frogs and in Mexico worms.

Traditionally chocolate is also considered an aphrodisiac. This probably originates from the time when chocolate was scarce and hence expensive. It contains phenylethylamine, related in structure to the so-called neuro-transmitters, but it is broken down before it reaches the brain. In addition there are minimal quantities of caffeine, thebromine and anadomine. None of these ingredients can explain the reviving effect of chocolate. Women are supposed to experience a pacifying and hormone-calming effect, for example when sexually aroused.

Avocados, oysters, mussels and asparagus are also considered to be aphrodisiacs, and when they appear on the menu are meant to herald fireworks in bed. This hypothesis rests solely on the supposed similarity of these foods to genitalia, which can also be found in bananas, carrots, figs, peaches and coconuts. Avocados grow in pairs and are supposedly reminiscent of testicles. The durian is fruit the size of a football with spines, which grows on huge trees in South-East Asia. It has a distinctive flavour and is held to be aphrodisiac. As a Malay proverb puts it: 'When the durians are down, the sarongs are up.'

Training apparatus

In the 1920s various theories were developed on the anatomy and physiology of the erection; drive rods and Magdeburg hemispheres were used as analogies. Therapeutically, however, things did not advance beyond the prescription of testosterone preparations. In the Dutch *Journal of Sexology* of December 1994 there is description of how papaverine and yohimbine was already in use in 1921 in the treatment of men with erection problems. The two substances, which were already believed to improve erection quality, were combined by a German researcher to form PYT (papaverine-yohimbine-tartrate).

Extensive animal research was carried out on this compound. According to the researcher tomcats displayed 'typical on-heat behaviour' after systematic administration, while in anaesthetized rats 'maximum vasodilation in the pelvis minor' was observed. It was also established what doses were fatal to a cat, a frog, a rabbit and a mouse. Male impotence cost the lives of so many animals! Without their knowledge, male syphilis patients became the first human guinea pigs: these were the days before committees on medical research ethics. The results of the pilot study were never published.

From 1940 to 1960, convinced that the traditional psychotherapeutic approach sometimes had no effect, the English psychiatrists Russell and Loewenstein used so-called coitus-training apparatus, with which the penis could be supported, enabling the man to have intercourse without an erection. The apparatus had an eye bolt with a rotatable link so that everything could be fastened as high as possible under the scrotum. In tightening the bolts care had to be taken that the pubic hairs were not trapped. The other end was placed around the penis in such a way that the scrotum could hang freely, but the glans could at the same time rest in a kind of ring, which was made of ebony and had five metal plates in the inside.

The theory was that the acidity and moisture level of the penis could be raised by an electric current, which would provide an effective stimulus. The purpose of this apparatus was to break the vicious circle of fear of failure and impotence, since it was evident even at that time

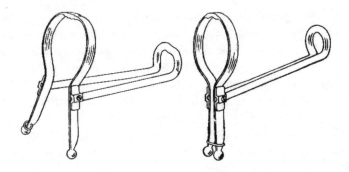

Coital training apparatus designed by psychiatrists in 1947.

that certain men were not motivated to undergo any kind of talking therapy.

A different, but to some extent comparable solution is the artificial penis, to which some women have an aversion. The use of a dildo – the exotic term for an artificial penis – is as old as mankind. In the nineteenth century they sold like hot cakes in all European capitals: clay, paper, wax – every kind of raw material was tried. In using such an aid one must of course observe strict hygiene, and the use of a lubricant is sensible. With an artificial penis full penetration is not necessary, and may even be undesirable.

High-tech: Old wine in new bottles

In the last decade urological interest in ED has increased spectacularly. This is a positive development for various reasons: for instance, more attention has been paid to the sexual consequences of operations. It has also become apparent that physical abnormalities are more frequently involved than had been traditionally assumed by sexology. In addition, both the diagnostic and therapeutic options in dealing with impotence have greatly increased.

On 25 June 1980 the French cardiovascular surgeon Ronald Virag discovered by accident that direct administration of papaverine into the penis could cause an erection, but he only published on the subject in *The Lancet* in 1982. Since the 1960s papaverine had been used in surgical procedures to keep the two blood vessels to be stitched together as wide open as possible: in other words, it is an established drug. Like opium, it is made from the poppyhead, but is completely non-addictive. During a cardiovascular surgical procedure Virag accidentally injected papaverine into the wrong vessel, inflicting an extremely long-lasting post-operative erection on the patient.

In fact, as long ago as the Second World War, the penis was used by military surgeons to transfuse large quantities of blood into soldiers in deep shock (because the relevant veins could no longer be seen or felt, it was sometimes impossible to insert a drip into the arm of patients in shock). However, if the blood flow was too fast, it resulted in an erection. Therefore injection therapy (in which the man injects himself in the penis with a vasodilatory drug) originates from the link established between a wartime procedure and a 'slip' during an operation.

In 1983 the world of urology was alarmed by a talk on this subject by the eccentric British professor Giles Brindley at the American Conference of Urologists in Las Vegas. He was conducting research into the effects of intrapenile administration of phentolamine, like papaverine a vasodilatory medication, but one that acted in a different way. Usually speakers at such a gathering are neatly dressed, that is, in suit and tie, but Professor Brindley appeared in shorts and sneakers. He talked about the results of his research, but after a quarter of an hour he interrupted the talk by announcing that he was getting a hard-on. The audience were shocked, not least because he went on to drop his shorts giving those at the front a close-up view and inviting them to feel it . . . He told us that he had injected himself before giving his presentation. An unforgettable, penetrating performance!

A prostaglandin or a combination of papaverine and phentolamine can be used for self-injection. This combination was officially registered for intercavernosal use in 1992 under the brand name Androskat. The dosage for treatment depends on the cause of the impotence. The effect is virtually immediate, or takes at most between fifteen minutes and half an hour. Depending on the firmness and duration of the erection, the dose should be adjusted step by step. A slow increase is preferable, and this is usually done in consultation with the urologist in charge of the case. In general the aim is to achieve an erection lasting between one and two hours. Injecting more than twice a week is not advisable, since this can cause sclerosis.

Penile injections can occasionally cause a long-lasting, usually painful erection (priapism). The blood is as it were trapped in the erectile tissue compartments, and is no longer replaced by new blood. As a result oxygen deficiency occurs and if action is not taken in time this is followed by morbidity in the erectile tissue. A faulty technique can result in a subcutaneous injection, and there will often be visible haemorrhaging; the same can occur in a patient taking blood-thinning medication. Caution must be used with patients suffering from cataracts or ailments in which an acute drop in blood pressure can be dangerous, for example shortly after a heart attack. Worldwide not only papaverine, phentolamine and prostaglandin EI, but also moxysylyte (especially in France), vasoactive intestinal polypeptide (VIP), ketanserin, calcitonin gene-related peptide and chlorpromazine are used.

Intracavernosal
injection.

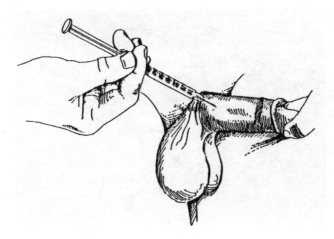

Papaverine was naturally also tested on women . . . Gynaecologists
were keen to try injections into the labia minora (specifically, the bulbus
vestibulum) with anorgasmic women, in the hope of producing at least
some 'moistening effect'. Attempts failed, and no orgasms resulted.

The vacuum pump

A more or less natural erection can be simulated not only by the implantation of an erection prosthesis, but also by the use of a so-called
vacuum pump in combination with a penile constriction ring. Down
the ages the constriction ring has been used a sex aid. Four hundred
years ago in Japan penile rings belonged in so-called love boxes and
Bedouins used the dried eyelashes of goats to make them. It was
thought that the lashes would provide extra stimulus during intercourse and arouse the woman sexually. Such rings are still available in
sex shops.

Vacuum apparatus has been on the market for almost a hundred
years. Zabludowsky's version is described in *Manual of the Sexual
Sciences* (1912) by the German psychiatrist Albert Moll. Until recently
vacuum erection apparatus attracted almost no attention in medical
circles, but plenty from the owners of sex shops, where it is on sale
even today.

The modern vacuum apparatus consists of a cylinder, a pump and
constriction band or ring. A true vacuum (with zero air pressure) is fortunately never achieved, since if it were the pump would be entirely
filled with a bleeding penis. Actually a better name would be underpressure apparatus. The cylinder, closed at one end, is slid over the
penis, open end first, and pushed against the pubic bone to form an

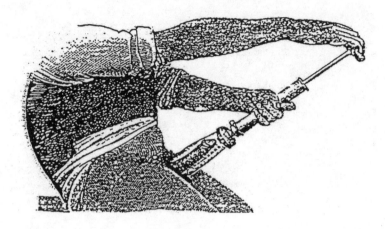

airtight seal. It is sometimes useful to cut away the pubic hair at the base of the penis. At the closed end the cylinder is connected to the pump, which creates underpressure in the cylinder, so that blood is sucked towards the erectile tissue and an erection is created. The required pressure is 120 millibars, which is the pressure in the erectile tissue compartments in erection. In reality, however, more is needed. When the penis is sufficiently erect, the ring, which was previously placed round the base of the cylinder, is rolled down, so that the outflow of blood from the erectile tissue compartments is impeded. At that moment some blood always leaks away, causing a proportionately large loss of pressure. This is why an underpressure of 200 millibars must be built up. Once the constriction ring is in place, blood can no longer leak out of the erectile tissue compartments. The ring has an indentation on its underside to avoid the urethra being squeezed completely shut, impeding ejaculation. The ring must remain in place no longer than 30 minutes and naturally one must not sleep with it on.

Because of the accumulation of blood the penis may turn slightly blue. Sometimes there are small pinpoint haemorrhages, and the penis may feel cold. 'It was like making love to an iceberg,' as one woman put it. The base of the penis may also wobble, thus sometimes complicating insertion. It goes without saying that the use of a vacuum apparatus during intercourse stands or falls with the presence of a sympathetic and understanding woman, who does not make excessive aesthetic demands on the man's phallus.

The vacuum pump with a rubber constriction ring at the base.

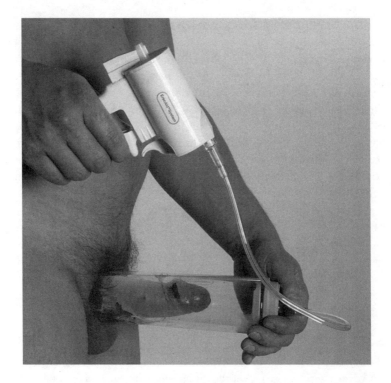

Inspired by the penis bone

The first operation to insert a penis prosthesis took place in 1936. In order to reconstruct a male member amputated in a trauma, the plastic surgeon Bogoras implanted a section of rib cartilage, prompted by his observation of the presence of a penis bone in many male mammals. The human penis is rather an odd man out, since that of numerous other mammals contains such a bone, called a *baculum*. These include the whale, the dolphin, the walrus, the otter, the bear, the marten, the badger, the squirrel, the wolf, the dog and the monkey. In some species, for example in the spider monkey, there is also a section of bone or cartilage in the clitoris.

In 1951 Bett wrote an extensive article on the penis bone. In the whale the bone is some 2 metres long, with a circumference of 40 cm at the base. Further up the evolutionary ladder it becomes smaller: in the walrus it is only just over 50 cm and in the monkey it measures only between 1 and 2 cm. Up to now there are no indications that homo sapiens ever possessed such a bone. The position and shape of the bone vary from animal to animal. In the dog, for example, it forms a channel for the urethra, while in the bear and the wolf the baculum is indispensable for mating. The baculum may have many different kinds of shape. In the racoon, for example, it is s-shaped and in the bat it is forked. In the squirrel there is a sharp hook attached, which according to some experts is designed to perforate the hymen. Others believe that the hook is designed to remove so-call mating plugs. A mating plug consists of a sticky residue of sperm allowing the vagina of the female squirrel to be temporarily 'sealed' in order to prevent sperm donation by another male. In the otter the penis bone is characterized by extreme hardness, though healed penis fractures have been observed in these creatures. When male otters fight each other, they target their opponent's penis with their powerful jaws and sharp teeth, and often succeed in breaking the baculum!

The penis bone also occasionally crops up in literature. Henry Miller, the first serious modern writer to give an honest account of his turbulent love life, mentions it in *Tropic of Cancer*, in his colourful style:

> O Tania, where now is that warm cunt of yours, those fat, heavy garters, those soft, bulging thighs? There is a bone in my prick six inches long. I will ream out every wrinkle in your cunt, Tania, big with seed . . . I shoot hot bolts into you, Tania, I make your ovaries incandescent. Your Sylvester is a little jealous now? He feels something, does he? He feels the remnants of my big prick. I have set the shores a little wider. I have ironed out the wrinkles. After me you can take on stallions, bulls, rams, drakes, St. Bernards.

This fantasy is not a degradation of women, far from it. It is modern man's painfully transparent anxiety: sexual envy and fear of having too small a penis.

The use of genuine rib cartilage as a penis prosthesis proved inadequate in the long term: the material was eventually reabsorbed by the body. For this reason synthetic prostheses were developed in the 1950s. To begin with these were inserted in the penis, but outside the erectile tissue compartments. This had in fact been tried thousands of years previously in China: with chicken bones. The problem was that in time

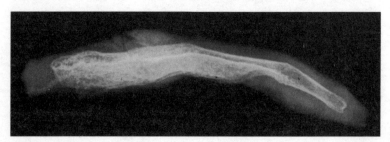

x-ray photo of a
dog's baculum.

The inflatable erection prosthesis.

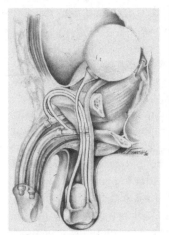
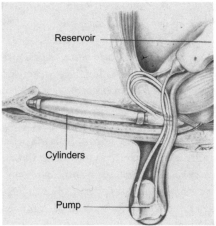

the chicken bone bored through the skin, and initially the same thing happened with the subcutaneously inserted prostheses. For that reason the technique was modified; in 1960 Beheri described the operating technique still current today in which two plastic cylinders, which may or may not be inflatable, are placed in the erectile tissue compartments and as it were fill them; this procedure entails the permanent loss of the spongiform erectile tissue.

The implanting of a prosthetic is an irrevocable step, since it involves the sacrificing of the penis's own capacity to swell. Even given optimum information it is often difficult for patients and their partners to imagine in advance what living with a penile prosthesis will be like. Talking to a patient who has already been through a similar procedure – usually a very effective way of briefing patients – is generally not feasible, often due in large part to false modesty on both sides. In this way things remain veiled in secrecy. We find this in the novel *The Story of R* (1990) by the Italian writer Gaia Servadio, in which her main character, a rich businesswoman, tells her adored young lover the following about a penile prosthesis:

'I shouldn't be telling you these things, but the Baron's just come back from Bulgaria where he had plastic surgery done to his . . . yes, well, eh, you know what I'm talking about! A small internal pump so that with a bit of manipulation, he can get it up. Apparently it's a painful operation, but many people have it done. I mean, what is one to do? When a man's reached the age of seventy, he knows everything there is to know about sex, but he can't do anything about it any more. For women it's different, eh?'

'But once the pump's been inserted, what can a man do? Can he still have orgasms?'

Well, that is possible, since experiencing an orgasm is not in itself dependent on an erection. Experience shows, though, that most men are very attached to an orgasm with an erect penis. As regards the quality of orgasm, this is never reduced after the implantation of a prosthesis.

There are various kinds of prosthesis on the market. The semi-rigid type consists of two flexible plastic cylinders, one of which is placed in each erectile tissue compartment. For aesthetic reasons it is sensible to carry out a circumcision at the same time. After implantation the penis is constantly in an erect state, but its flexibility is such that it can be hidden under clothing. It could be compared to the bendability of an old-fashioned desk lamp. The much more expensive inflatable prosthesis has the advantage that the penis remains flaccid when 'at rest', and that a natural erection is simulated. The prosthesis comprises two inflatable cylinders. As with the semi-rigid prosthesis, the cylinders are placed in the erectile tissue compartments. The length of the cylinders is not decided until the operation is in progress, and this requires great precision. If they are too long there is a danger that the casing of the erectile tissue compartment will be perforated. If they are too short the so-called 'Concorde phenomenon' may occur, that is, the glans may droop during an erection. The cylinders in the erectile tissue compartments are linked to a pump in the scrotum and with a fluid reservoir in the abdominal cavity. When an erection is required, the cylinders can be filled with fluid by squeezing the pump. Some dexterity is required to operate the prosthesis. Scientific research has shown that penile prostheses cause few problems in daily life. In the case of semi-rigid prostheses it is not always possible to camouflage the penis properly, and for that reason tight swimming trunks are not recommended.

More than three-quarters of patients who have had an operation are satisfied. The principal reasons for dissatisfaction mentioned are the impossibility of intercourse (especially after implantation of a semi-rigid prosthesis) and the absence of an orgasm. Almost all patients would have the operation again. This obviously means that even a defective restitution of the capacity for erection can be seen as a successful restoration of the battered sense of male self-esteem.

It is important to gain a clear picture before the operation of the pattern of expectations of both the patient and his partner. This is not work for a urologist alone, and preferably there should always be a sexologist involved. Unfortunately it does sometimes transpire that it would have been better if a patient had not had the operation. A practical example: a 50-year-old man had had impotence problems for a considerable time. Based on the evidence of various tests the urologist was convinced that these were psychological in origin, and consequently referred the patient to a sexologist. It soon became apparent that the man involved had a rather unhappy prehistory. He married young, but divorced a few years later and shortly afterwards entered into a homosexual relationship. Later he nevertheless felt more attracted to women. After having led a rather wild life up to then, things became calmer. He curbed his excessive drinking and married a somewhat older woman. Unfortunately this relationship also went wrong: his wife fell in love with a member of the choir at the church they had joined, and the marriage foundered.

The patient, undeterred, embarked on a new relationship, but now unfortunately his penis let him down. And what happened? The sexologist he consulted could not help him, but referred him back to the urologist with the request that he be taught to give himself intrapenile injections. That soon proved a failure: haemorrhages, complaints of pain, and so on. A vacuum pump did not help. Only after a great deal of humming and hawing was the patient prepared to return to the sexologist, and his new partner refused to accompany him. Finally, at the patient's insistence, it was decided to implant a prosthesis, the semi-rigid type, since the urologist felt the patient was probably not dextrous enough to operate an inflatable prosthesis, and also to reduce costs (since hospitals have to keep within budget). Fortunately the procedure was completed without complications.

However, during a follow-up check the patient expressed his dissatisfaction at the final outcome of the operation. He did not tell his daughter about the operation and said that he saw her looking at his crotch while he was holding his granddaughter on his lap. He was convinced that his daughter saw his 'erect' penis and hence had started avoiding him. This story is hard to argue with, and might be grounds for discontinuing the implantation of semi-rigid prostheses.

Viagra

Strange as it may seem, the medicine that broke all sales records was a fluke. At the pharmaceuticals group Pfizer researchers were looking for a new medication for cardiovascular disease. One substance reviewed was sildenafil, the active component of the Viagra pill. There was considerable hope that it would be possible to use it to combat chest pains (angina pectoris), but in clinical tests in the 1990s the drug seemed to be a flop. Researchers detected little of the intended effect on the heart and the group saw little hope of a return on its investment. Then, strangely enough, reports came in from test subjects of unforeseen, but definitely pleasant side-effects. The strength of the drug Viagra lay not in the ribcage, but in the penis: long-lasting, hard erections and more stamina in lovemaking. A number of test subjects flatly refused to return their supply of the drug at the end of the research period and one of them even satisfied his need by breaking into the research lab. It slowly began to dawn on those concerned that with sildenafil the solution to a problem affecting men all over the world had fallen into their lap.

Once the desire has been awakened and the stage of foreplay is reached, an erection pill can do its work. Between twenty and 30 minutes after the drug has been taken the erection-causing action kicks in. How do sildenafil and the more modern PDE5 inhibitors work? With the right mood and in the right circumstances nerve impulses from the brain stimulate the production of cyclic guanosine monophosphate (CGMP) in the penis. As a result the smooth muscle cells of the spongiform network in the erectile tissue compartments relax. (When the penis is flaccid, the smooth muscle cells are on the contrary taut.) The penis finds rest only in erection, in sex and, for by far the longest periods, each night during REM sleep.

When CGMP is released into the erectile tissue compartments there is a dilation of the arteries, and more blood flows in. At the same time the increasing volume of blood forces the exiting veins shut, retaining blood in the penis and causing an erection.

The enzyme phosphodiesterase 5 (PDE5) breaks down CGMP, so that the erection is not maintained and the blood flows away as fast as it enters. This the point at which PDE5 inhibitors like sildenafil (Viagra), vardenafil (Levitra) and tadalafil (Cialis) help by neutralizing the erection killer phosphodiestarase 5. Cialis has the longer effect, 36 hours, and is also called 'the weekend pill', offering the advantage that intercourse does not have to happen soon after taking the pill: one can wait until Saturday or even Sunday – an important consideration, knowing that many women dislike making love to order. PDE5 inhibitors protect CGMP, then, so that blood remains longer in the erectile tissue compartments. PDE5 inhibitors act not only in the penis, but also in varying degrees in the other PDE receptors. By 2007 twelve of these had been identified. The most common side-effects of PDE5 inhibitors are headache, a reddish complexion, a full feeling in the stomach region, a bluish haze in front of the eyes, dizziness and skin rashes. In these locations PDE inhibitors with a different number have been pinpointed. The PDE5 inhibitors, for example, act to a minor extent on the PDE6 receptors in the retina. In addition it is important that PDE5 inhibitors should not be taken at the same time as medication containing nitrate; this can cause sharp drops in blood pressure. Since 2006 sildenafil has had one other official use: the drug can lower blood pressure in the pulmonary circulation. Raised blood pressure in the blood vessels of the lung is life-threatening and sometimes very difficult to treat.

At the end of 2006 banner headlines announced that British doctors had saved the life of a premature baby with Viagra. The doctors administered the drug to a little boy, who at birth weighed only 780 g and was struggling with one non-functioning lung. The medication opened tiny blood vessels in his lungs, allowing oxygen to be absorbed by his blood in spite of this. The parents of baby Lewis, who had been born in August 2006, feared for his life and had even prepared for the funeral – but in December they were able to take him home!

PDE5 inhibitors are registered only for men with erection problems. Studies in women were inconclusive and did not finally result in registration. Female sexual problems tend to be more complicated and consist of symptoms that are hard to quantify. PDE5 inhibitors have a salutary effect on men's minds and perhaps also on their relationships with women, as was maintained by the actor Jack Nicholson in an interview with *Playboy* in 2004:

> Over the years I have heard many people, after ending a marriage or a relationship, say, 'I would never have left her if I could have said, without fear of shattering her entire existence, 'I just don't want sex anymore.' The relationship could have continued if I had been able to say, 'Fuck someone else if you want.' Everything would have been fine between us. Instead, the disinterest in sex that can come along becomes so intense that it can dominate the relationship. Viagra solves that. Once, twice a month – and regardless of what people tell you, that's enough – stimulate yourself with this pharmacological solution, go out there and tear Mom up, baby, and everything is fine. It could save many relationships.

Getting older

As the years go by most men notice that they sometimes have trouble in achieving an erection or maintaining it for long enough. Some conclude that this means they are finished as sexual beings, that they have reached the 'penopause'. Understandable, if one knows that many of them were brought up with the idea that sex is actually something like 'fertilizing', or at least being capable of it. The machine has to be in good order, or 'there's no point', as they put it.

Obviously every person reacts differently to growing older. Some cease to perform much physical activity somewhere between the ages of twenty and 30. For the present generation of heart surgeons it's nothing special to have to insert artificial coronary arteries in someone in their thirties. Others withdraw into a shell for years and then once they turn fifty emerge with great zest. Often it ends in disappointment. There are those who continue swimming, playing badminton or something similar as they have always done – perhaps not as fast at 50 as at twenty, but still keeping active. The same applies more or less to sexual activities. With the passing of the years all men have to rein themselves in a little, but not all at the same age and/or with the same consequences. Some men drop their sexual activities early, sometimes completely, sometimes in part. Others stay active until some illness more or less takes them by surprise and they have to keep themselves in check.

Some men associate sex with the battle against death. Because their organ refuses to 'stand up and fight' any longer, they are frightened of losing the battle. These men particularly are relieved when they hear from the lips of a specialist that the penis always becomes less rigid with the passing of time, and that it's more or less normal that their penis should let them down occasionally. They then usually forego artificial therapies. Their marriage no longer desperately needs consummating: the important thing was to know whether or not death was round the corner.

The physical manifestations of the penopause are often accompanied by brooding: the man starts reflecting on the life he has led up to then. What have I achieved of all the things I once dreamed of? I shall have to stay married to this woman till death do us part. Until my dying day I will never again see anything else but the same furniture, the same house, the same street. And until I retire I shall have to go on slogging away day after day at that stupid job of mine! The man at this stage is regularly ambushed by these kinds of reflections. He begins to wonder what the future has to offer him. Though he is still fertile, it is possible for a man to think that his potency is declining. In that case the occasional lovemaking session may go wrong.

Men should worry less about the fact that as they get older their penis occasionally goes on strike. But that's precisely the point. Often when it happens out of the blue the man starts worrying seriously, which in turn provokes fear of failure. Guilt ensues and the man concerned eventually comes to find lovemaking torture.

A fairy tale about ageing

When God had created the world and was about to fix the length of each creature's life, the ass came and asked, 'Lord, how long shall I live?' 'Thirty years,' replied God; 'does that content thee?' 'Ah, Lord,' answered the ass, 'that is a long time. Think of my painful existence! To carry heavy burdens from morning to night, to drag sacks of corn to the mill, that others may eat bread, to be cheered and refreshed with nothing but blows and kicks. Relieve me of a portion of this long time.' Then God had pity on him and relieved him of eighteen years. The ass went away comforted, and the dog appeared. 'How long wouldst thou like to live?' said God to him. 'Thirty years are too many for the ass, but thou wilt be satisfied with that.' 'Lord,' answered the dog, 'is that thy will? Consider how I shall have to run, my feet will never hold out so long, and when I have once lost my voice for barking, and my teeth for biting, what will be left for me to do but run from one corner to another and growl?' God saw that he was right, and released him from twelve years of life. Then came the monkey. 'Thou wilt certainly live thirty years willingly?' said the Lord to him. 'Thou hast no need to work as the ass and the dog have to do, and wilt always enjoy thyself.' 'Ah! Lord,' he answered, 'it may seem as if that were the case, but it is quite different. When it rains porridge I have no spoon. I am always obliged to play merry pranks, and make faces which force people to laugh, and if they give me an apple, and I bite into it, why it is sour! How often sadness hides itself behind mirth! I shall never be able to hold out for thirty years.' God was gracious and took off ten.

At last man appeared, joyous, healthy and vigorous, and begged God to appoint his time for him. 'Thirty years shalt thou live,' said the Lord. 'Is that enough for thee?' 'What a short time,' cried man, 'when I have built my house and my fire burns on my own hearth; when I have planted trees which blossom and bear fruit, and am just intending to enjoy my life, I am to die! O Lord, lengthen my time.' 'I will add to it the ass's eighteen years,' said God. 'That is not enough,' replied the man. 'Thou shalt also have the dog's twelve years.' 'Still too little!' 'Well, then,' said God, 'I will give thee the monkey's ten years also, but more thou shalt not have.' The man went away, but was not satisfied.

So man lives seventy years. The first thirty are his human years, which are soon gone; then is he healthy, merry, works with pleasure, and is glad of his life. Then follow the ass's eighteen years, when one burden after another is laid on him, he has to carry the corn which feeds others, and blows and kicks are the reward of his faithful services. Then come the dog's twelve years, when he lies in the corner, and growls and has no longer any teeth to bite with, and when this time is over the monkey's ten years form the end. Then man is weak-headed and foolish, does silly things, and becomes the jest of the children.

This fairy tale by the Brothers Grimm, written over a hundred years ago, expresses very succinctly a view of older people that is current even today. Very many young people assume that the above-mentioned stupid old monkeys no longer indulge in sexual activities. Place 'old' in front of some of the slang words for penis, and the insult stings even more. Being called a 'prick' is bad enough, but an 'old prick', one that no longer works, is far worse. What man does not dread the moment when his penis leaves him in the lurch once and for all?

Growing old has been compared to a game of chess, in which pieces are eventually lost, though certain strong pieces still control the board and can even engineer a powerful new position. But every chess player knows what the loss of the queen means in a game. The power of the queen is a very good analogy for the meaning of eroticism in a human life. In fact, it is not the loss of sexual performance, but the loss of the erotic dimension that generates most apprehension in confronting old age. Men can sometimes exorcize that fear, for example, through singing with their comrades. I was once given, by an anaesthetist friend of mine with greying temples, who had served as a doctor during his military service, the words of a song sung by British officers in the mess in the evenings. They are as follows:

Your spooning days are over
Your pilot light is out
What used to be your sex appeal
Is now your water spout

You used to be embarrassed
To make the thing behave
For every bloody morning it
Stood up to watch you shave
But now that you are growing old
It sure gives you the blues
To see the thing hang down your leg
And watch you shine your shoes

One thing remains: with the passing of the years the frequency of sexual activity declines. The Rotterdam physiologist and sexologist Koos Slob presented the following figures based on various surveys: 84 per cent of men in their fifties, 67 per cent of those in their sixties, 43 per cent of septuagenarians and 16 per cent of octogenarians are sexually active.

For women the percentages are 76 per cent (51–60), 40 per cent (61–70) and 7 per cent (71–80) respectively. No survey information is available for women over 80. There are certainly great individual differences. The decline in later years is shown to be least in those most active at a young age.

Until quite recently experts believed that ED later in life was almost always the result of arteriosclerosis. There are also indications that the stiffness of the penis declines as one gets older as a result of a change in composition of both the erectile tissue compartments and the stiff capsule of connective tissue surrounding them, which plays an important part in retaining blood. It is anyway generally true that muscles, tendons and articular capsules grow thinner with age and lose their elasticity, and the loss of elasticity in the erectile tissue compartments is actually the main reason why the penis becomes shorter as one gets older. Of course there are other factors that can affect potency in the elderly. Chronic medication dependency and diseases like diabetes mellitus are more prevalent. Joint calcification caused, for example, by rheumatism, may cause pain and restrict movement, impeding intercourse. And although heart attacks and strokes need not automatically lead to problems in lovemaking the patient and his partner are understandably often frightened of a recurrence.

After a heart attack many men don't dare ask their doctor for advice about their sex lives. For example, what exactly does 'taking it easy' mean in this context? It may well be that a reduction in sexual activity will have an adverse effect on the patient's condition. It is understandable that men who have had a heart attack should be worried about putting too much strain on their heart, but heart patients can have a perfectly satisfying sex life without putting themselves at risk. Driving in heavy traffic, playing with a grandchild or having a heated discussion put more pressure on the heart than sexual intercourse. Research into the incidence of heart attacks during intercourse revealed that when these occurred they were almost always related to an extramarital affair, making such affairs particularly inadvisable for heart patients.

Set in one's ways

'Getting stuck in a rut' as one gets older is the theme of Guy de Maupassant's story 'Set in One's Ways' ('La Rouille'), which describes how Monsieur and Madame de Courville finally fail to get the old Baron Hector Gontran de Coutelier to marry Berthe Vilers. To begin with the baron is very enthusiastic about the proposed bride-to-be, and she accompanies him on many hunting parties, but when after a while he is asked straight out if he wants to marry her, he appears dumbstruck. Weeks later he announces to Monsieur de Courville that he does not wish to pursue the proposed marriage and months later confesses once and for all that he is impotent. The baron had decided first to go to Paris and had visited several ladies of loose morals, none of whom had been able to provoke an erection. Next he tried all kinds of piquant dishes, which did nothing but upset his stomach. He draws his conclusions and makes his confession. As he listens, Monsieur de Courville has great difficulty in not bursting out laughing, and on his return home he tells the story to his wife. She doesn't laugh, but listens attentively and when the story is over says the following: 'The baron is an idiot, my dear; he was afraid, that's all. I'll write to Berthe and tell her to come back straightaway . . . when a man loves his wife, you know, those things . . . always sort themselves out.'

The psychoanalyst Wilhelm Stekel (1868–1940), a breakaway pupil of Sigmund Freud's, takes the view that under certain circumstances the potency of older people can improve. According to Stekel, the peak of a man's potency depends not on age, but on the sexual 'object' available to him. In one's youth the sexual urge is generally stronger and more tempestuous. The man is less concerned about the soulmate who can satisfy him fully, than with 'the bit of skirt' that meets his taste and his daily needs. According to Stekel that is why many younger men may frequent prostitutes and as they grow older stop. In his view, in maturity, as desire becomes more refined, love becomes increasingly something 'in the head', which is why under certain circumstances potency can be even greater. Stekel believes that only in a sexually harmonious marriage, with mutual understanding between the partners, can the wife respond to the 'refined taste' and the 'intellectual desire'. The man must show himself capable of bringing about a 'spiritualization' of the marriage . . .

He illustrates this with the story of an elderly painter. His considerably younger wife is described by Stekel as a strikingly intelligent, 'Juno-esque' lady of amazing beauty. The man has been impotent for twenty years. To begin with he still had erections, but these invariably disappeared the moment his wife approached. For the last ten years he has had no erections at all, not even in the mornings. In addition he suffers from nocturnal panic attacks, and is afraid of developing a heart complaint. The man's behaviour is unpredictable and he often loses his self-control. These days his wife is only happy when he is away. He blames his wife:

> Do you know, doctor, even when I was young I often couldn't perform normal intercourse. There always has to be an element

of danger for me to perform well. You may laugh! I've never really been potent in bed, only with my wife when we were first married. But if I could throw some girl into a corner, on the floor or onto the sofa, then it was always terrific.

His wife had fallen in love with him because she admired his paintings so much. She was his pupil, but gave up painting when they got married. When she took up painting again, he realized that he really didn't care for her mediocre work. Subsequently his wife began criticizing his paintings, and took the side of an art critic who had attacked his work:

'Was that before your impotence?' asks Stekel.
'Wait a moment, I remember the exact date of the exhibition. And the date of my first disgrace, it was my wife's birthday, and we were in Semmering . . . Of course. The disgrace befell me a few months later.'

During the course of psychoanalysis his wife died. Two weeks later he raped his hunchbacked cook. A few months later he dismissed the cook and fell in love with a young pupil, who idolized him, and with whom he proves quite potent enough to be able to make love in the normal way in bed . . . .
Stekel regards this case as an example of the dichotomy between animal and 'spiritualized' love The man undoubtedly harboured brutal and possessive sexual desires from an early age, but his sexual potency failed him when his wife denied him her 'spiritual' admiration, thus turning into a 'bit of skirt', whom he would most like to fling onto the sofa.

Priapism

Priapism is a totally different affliction of the penis. It is the medical term for a usually painful erection lasting longer than three hours, with a complete absence of any sexual arousal.
In Graeco-Roman mythology Priapus is one of the lesser gods, of fertility, viticulture, gardening, beekeeping, etc. He is usually depicted with a gigantic phallus, and originated from Asia Minor. In the eyes of more educated Romans, Priapus was a figure of fun. He was imported from Greece in the first century by Roman practitioners of lighter verse.
Almost always he is pictured as a scarecrow and a deterrent to thieves keeping watch over a patch of land growing some vegetables and fruit and his coloured image is carved from a rough piece of wood. He is considered to be a connoisseur of the erotic, whose rough appearance is echoed in his forthright language, and who is immensely proud

of his phallus. The *Carmina Priapea*, a collection of nearly a hundred obscene erotic poems from AD 100, are quite explicit about Priapus' life and works.

The Priapus of the *Priapea* is a sexual glutton, a genuine Roman macho, who penetrates wherever he can. His sexuality is violent and unfeeling and some people have seen this as typical of the Roman male from the time of Nero:

> Take heed: a boy behind, a girl in front I'll take.
> For bearded men who steal, remains a third ordeal.

Briefly summarized, that is the standard penalty for theft from Priapus' garden or orchard. Depending on whether the offender is a woman, a man or a boy, they are threatened with vaginal, oral or anal rape. Priapus is also offered sacrifices in the poems, which are not only about crude sex. In one a dancer dedicates her tambourine and castanets to Priapus, expressing the hope that her audience will stay as enthusiastic as Priapus himself. Another promiscuous woman offers a generous number of wooden penises, one for every man she has 'serviced' the night before.

Priapism may occur as a side-effect of self-injection in the penis, but can also be the result of leukaemia, malignant tumours in the lower abdomen, the use of certain drugs and also sickle-cell anaemia, a hereditary disease affecting mainly non-white populations living in or originating historically from tropical or subtropical malarial regions. In this condition the red blood cells are more or less deformed, assuming a sickle shape, so that blood-clotting can quite easily occur, particularly when the flow speed is reduced. An instance of reduced flow is the state of erection, especially in sometimes 50-minute-long nocturnal erections. Young men with sickle-cell anaemia are prone to priapism. Treatment consists of the injection of a vascular constrictive medication directly into the penis. If that doesn't help, an operation is necessary, in which a kind of bypass is constructed from the penis to an inguinal vein, allowing the accumulated blood to drain away uninterrupted. There are many variants: if an operation also fails to bring about flaccidity the erectile tissue compartments will fill up with connective tissue, giving them a wooden feel.

This happened to one of our patients not so long ago: after taking medication for depression a man, not yet 40, developed priapism. Unfortunately it emerged that that not all doctors are equally up to date on the treatment of priapism: it is necessary to act as soon as possible after such an erection, which is often very painful, and preferably within six hours. He was dismissed by his doctor, who did not take the trouble to consult a specialist. Eventually the patient submitted a claim to his GP's insurance company. However, damages had never been paid in the Netherlands in such a case, so that the patient's lawyer sought advice from colleagues abroad. He found that in the United States about 200,000 euros would be paid out. The patient received less than a tenth of that . . .

The crooked penis

The name of Marquis François Gigot de la Peyronie, personal physican to King Louis xv, is linked to a most unusual abnormality of the penis. Peyronie's disease indicates a crooked erect penis caused by excessive connective tissue formation in the wall of the erectile tissue compartment. At the point affected a hardening develops and elasticity is lost, hence causing crookedness in the erect position. The ailment is common, affecting an estimated 3.6 per cent of all adult males, and in most cases the onset is around the age of fifty. Approximately 20 per cent also suffer from connective tissue formation in and around tendon sheaths in the palm (Dupuytren's disease), and the occasional one has problems on the sole of the foot. The cause of Peyronie's disease is an abnormal inflammatory reaction in and under the capsule around the erectile tissue compartments, virtually always on the top, which means that the crooked position in the vast majority of cases is towards the abdomen.

A crooked penis may also be the result of a congenital asymmetry of the erectile tissue compartments, in which case the bend is towards the ground or sideways. The estimated incidence of congenital crookedness is six per thousand male babies.

Peyronie's disease is not an easy ailment to go public with, or a suitable conversation topic at parties. Consequently the patient often thinks that he has a 'unique' malady, whereas it is something run-of-the-mill. Its manifestations are pain, insufficient hardness of erection or an awkward *intromissio vaginalis*, in which the penis can be inserted only with great difficulty. Above all a member shaped like a boomerang can make sex very painful for the woman, though many women appeared to be intrigued by a crooked penis.

The cause of Peyronie's disease is still unknown. Mainly on the basis of the existence of related ailments thinking tends to favour abnormal genes, for which scientists are at present searching. As regards treatment, the Marquis de la Peyronie sent his patients to Barega, a spa in the Pyrenees. Not such a bad cure, when one knows that 40 per cent of patients will show some improvement in due course. However, the restoration of a ramrod-stiff penis will be out of the question for the patient concerned. Over the years more than a hundred non-operative

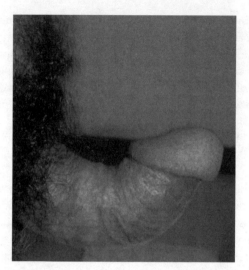

Crooked position in Peyronie's disease.

treatments have been described in the literature. That in itself says enough: not a single one has been convincingly proved to produce a cure.

If a year after the onset of the disease there is still serious crooked-ness, then provided the complaints of pain have ceased, there is good reason for an operation to correct the crookedness. Problems of rigid-ity are not solved by an operation, but problems with intercourse can be alleviated. The most frequently mentioned problem is that the penis regularly 'flops out' while the patient is thrusting. There are two different operations. In one the hard area is cut away and the defect created is covered with tissue taken from elsewhere or with synthetic material. In the other surgical technique the hard area is left untouched, and instead the operation takes place on the healthy side, where the penis is pulled back into line by the cutting out of small elliptical sections of wall or by a series of so-called reef knots. The main snag is that the penis may be shortened slightly, in addition to the shortening caused by the disease. The advantage is that there is no chance of developing ED. In contrast to the first operation, where the diseased tissue is removed, the malady is here treated with stitches on the healthy side.

Hypospadia

Hypospadia is a condition in which the opening of the urethra – which is normally at the top of the glans – is located on the underside, the shaft of the penis or even in the scrotum. In addition the foreskin on the underside of the glans is missing, and the erect penis is sometimes also bent. Approximately 1 in 300 males is born with this abnormality. The cause of hypospadia is very probably a relative testosterone deficiency between the sixth and thirteenth week of pregnancy.

To enable a patient to urinate standing up and function normally sexually, the end of the urethra must be reconstructed and the penis stretched. In the past children with this condition were not operated on until they were older, but today urologists prefer to perform the operation before the child enters its third year, thus limiting the psychological trauma of hospital admission as far as possible. For the manufacture of a new section of urethra use is made of the inner leaf of the foreskin. If the foreskin has already been removed, one can also use mucous membrane from the cheek or lip. Scars, the relatively short penis length and the abnormal shape of the glans mean that some boys, particularly in their adolescence, are not really satisfied with the result of the operation. The urologists who operated on them usually are, but they know that their options will always be limited. Doctors can't really improve on the existing organ. It is important to make it quite clear to patients that correction of hypospadia will not lengthen the penis. Adolescents or adults complaining of too small a penis in particular should be offered help by a sexologist.

A very special form of hypospadia is *mika*. As an initiation ritual at the onset of puberty, the male inhabitants of the island of Mangaia in the Pacific have their urethra split open from the tip to the scrotum with a narrow incision. It is no accident that *mika* means 'the terrible ritual'. The procedure prevents semen from finding its way into the vagina during intercourse – a crude form of contraception! Australian Aborigines, as it happens, once had the same custom.

As a last resort in the event of several failed urethra operations, urologists sometimes go a step further by relocating the outlet of the urethra between the scrotum and the anus. Men who have had this treatment are therefore obliged to urinate in female fashion, namely squatting.

Phimosis and circumcision

A completely different but common ailment of the penis is phimosis, contraction of the foreskin. The only reason for operating on the foreskin is a lasting contraction that leads to problems. Virtually all newborn baby boys have a slight degree of phimosis with some adhesion, which almost always disappears spontaneously. Actually the term adhesion is incorrect: what is actually meant is that in the prenatal development of the sex organ the separation of the foreskin is not yet complete, and continues after birth. In only 4 per cent of newborn males can the foreskin be fully retracted, after six months the figure is 15 per cent, and at one year approximately half.

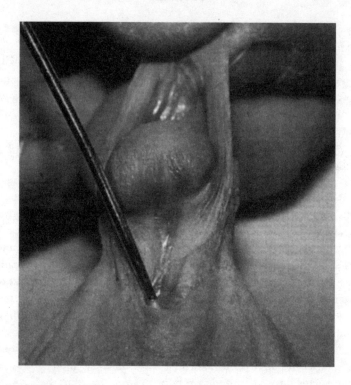

Hypospadia.

With phimosis, urine and smegma can accumulate between the glans and the inner leaf, causing an inflammation. Still, an operation is by no means always necessary, since it is usually possible to slide the foreskin back over the glans and to slide it back after applying some Vaseline, though using force must be avoided at all costs! If careful retraction takes place with some regularity, the aperture will become wide enough. If retraction, whether or not in combination with a corticoid cream, is unsuccessful, there is some reason for circumcision, but not otherwise.

In Western Europe when someone does something odd or deviant, he or she may be considered deranged and ignored, punished or treated. When a large number of people do something odd or deviant, it is called 'culture'. That also applies to ritual or religious circumcision. Jews and Muslims do it from religious conviction and some men even on aesthetic grounds (have you ever seen a foreskin in a porn movie?). Circumcision is a strange phenomenon but it is by no means as innocent as is often thought. To make the point, let's begin with a disastrous story from the Netherlands. In 2002 a young Moroccan boy underwent the 'standard' procedure. The operation was carried out by an ex-GP, supervised by a urologist, and in the course of it use was made of an 'electric' knife. Unfortunately it turned out that the operators had insufficient knowledge of the potential hazards of electro-surgical equipment. As a result the penis was partially coagulated, and went partly black. The three-year-old victim was virtually castrated and required extensive plastic surgery. Naturally the case had legal consequences, both criminal and civil.

Almost all urologists are familiar with the story of David Reimer. In his case too a large part of his penis was accidentally burned away when he was circumcised as a child. According to the psychologist John Money there was no problem, and the answer was simple. David was still so young that with some surgical cutting and patching and a large dose of hormones it was surely possible to turn David into a girl. What you've never known, you won't grieve over, the psychologist must have thought. And so it came to pass: David became Brenda. Money published a triumphant account of what he saw as his brilliant inspiration and its supposedly successful outcome. The truth was somewhat different: in 2004, at the age of 38, after an extended personal ordeal David/Brenda finally took his/her own life. The decision to turn a boy into a girl after a 'failed' circumcision is not unique. According to an article in the *National Enquirer* (22 October 1985), 200 babies die each year in America of complications arising from a circumcision.

Why circumcise? Opinions vary about the origin of ritual circumcision. The first indications of the existence of ritual circumcisions date back about five thousand years, when they formed an important element in heliolitic culture, in which sun worship was central. Nothing is known about the significance of circumcision at that time. In *The Eternity Machine*, Johannes and Peter Fiebag describe how gods once lived among men. Clearly these gods were susceptible to earthly maladies and required the humans who served them to be as pure as possible. Women with periods were not allowed to prepare meals and men too must be scrupulously clean. Circumcision was an obvious way of preventing dirt under the foreskin. The fear of pollution of the ancient gods fuelled the idea that the 'gods' may have been extraterrestrial. Via these primeval tales of hygienic gods the idea of circumcision crept into modern religions like Judaism and Islam. In this modern age, we tend to be sceptical of such mythologies.

Worldwide, then, circumcision takes place mainly on a ritual-religious basis. Shortly after the Second World War the Dutch Marxist A. Soep published an interesting ethnological study on this subject. He had forsaken Judaism, as is clear from the introduction to his very thorough, Marxism-based study, which is an indispensable reference work for specialists. Soep locates the first circumcision in ancient Egypt. The Egyptians originate from the countless nomadic tribes of Central and North Africa, and when they settled in the Nile delta they brought their cults and accompanying rituals with them. The Jews and Muslims in turn adopted ritual circumcision from the ancient Egyptians. In Soep's view the Egyptians saw circumcision mainly as a political-psychological symbol of superiority in respect of the uncircumcised nomadic peoples, including the Hebrews, who later formed the Jewish people.

According to the US NOCIRC website (www.nocirc.org), the oldest known depiction of a circumcision is an Egyptian print (Wellcome Institute Library), dating from 2420 BC. The print was found in the tomb of Anchmahor in Saqqara, from the sixth dynasty of the Old Kingdom. The circumcision is being carried out by an *hm-k3* (*ka* priest) and the relief consists of two scenes: in one, a boy is being held by the assistant of the *ka* priest, who is seated on the ground and is saying to the assistant: 'Hold him tight, so that he doesn't faint.' The assistant replies: 'I shall do as you say.' In the second scene the assistant is absent. The boy is still standing and places his hand on the head of the priest, who is sitting in front of him and rubbing something on his penis. The boy says: 'Rub it in very well.' The priest replies: 'I will make you comfortable.' Probably the ointment has anaesthetic properties, suggesting that the right-hand scene precedes the left-hand one.

Many anthropologists believe that circumcision is fundamentally a relic of human sacrifice. Sacrifices were made to the gods to be assured of their protection and beneficence. Complete devotion meant complete sacrifice. In order not to have to sacrifice a complete human being, a part of the principal organ, the organ of creation, a sacred force of nature, was sacrificed. With many peoples the removed foreskin was also burnt, as were human sacrifices. In this way the sacrificing of the foreskin became a symbol of the bond established between God and human beings. In Christianity circumcision was replaced by baptism, while Jews and Muslims have retained it. In Islam circumcision is seen mainly as a symbol of purity: a man must be circumcised before he can take part in religious ceremonies. In his book Soep devotes a great deal of attention to the various initiation ceremonies and the accompanying circumcision (and in some cultures clitoridectomy) in relation to the significance of puberty as the transition from a child to a sexually mature young man/woman – a kind of rebirth.

Even today all the sons of observant Muslims and Jews and the sons of tribes in Africa, Australia, Melanesia and Polynesia (except for New Zealand) are circumcised. In Polynesia the purpose of circumcision is to make the organ look clean and powerful, and because it is believed that with a circumcised penis one experiences a more powerful orgasm. Until 1990 virtually all baby boys were also circumcised in the United States shortly after birth. Jewish boys are circumcised when eight days old, Muslims as early as possible, but mostly before or during puberty. Worldwide, approximately one man in six is circumcised, and over 13 million circumcisions are carried out annually.

As pointed out above the tradition goes further back than the patriarch Abraham in the Bible, who at the age of 99 had himself circumcised with a sharp stone at God's command and then did the same to his son and all the males in his household. The story is told as follows in Genesis 17:10–14 and 23–27:

> This is my covenant, which ye shall keep, between me and you and thy seed after thee; Every man child among you shall be circumcised.
>
> And ye shall circumcise the flesh of your foreskin; and it shall be a token of the covenant betwixt me and you.
>
> And he that is eight days old shall be circumcised among you, every man child in your generations, he that is born in the house, or bought with money of any stranger, which is not of thy seed.
>
> He that is born in thy house, and he that is bought with thy money, must needs be circumcised: and my covenant shall be in your flesh for an everlasting covenant.
>
> And the uncircumcised man child whose flesh of his foreskin is not circumcised, that soul shall be cut off from his people; he hath broken my covenant.
>
> And Abraham took Ishmael his son, and all that were born in his house, and all that were bought with his money, every male among the men of Abraham's house; and circumcised the flesh of their foreskin the selfsame day, as God had said unto him.
>
> And Abraham ninety years old and nine, when he was circumcised in the flesh of his foreskin.
>
> And Ishmael his son was thirteen years old, when he was circumcised in the flesh of his foreskin.
>
> In the selfsame day was Abraham circumcised, and Ishmael his son.
>
> And all the men of his house, born in his house, and bought with money of the stranger, were circumcised with him.

In a monthly magazine on the religious upbringing of children, one theologian interpreted this as follows:

> Abraham becomes God's partner and so can no longer stay out of the firing line. The symbol of this is circumcision. The covenant cuts into Abraham's flesh, where he is most vulnerable, it 'sets a limit' to his manhood. Circumcision is a continual reminder of

the covenant with God. It symbolizes the fact that God's future will never be realized with male strength and potency alone.

Another wrote:

> The circumcision is not only the outward token of the covenant, but also means 'Be thou perfect', as God says to Abraham in Genesis 27:1. Literally, the Hebrew word translated as 'perfect' means: complete, all of a piece, whole. Not that Abraham is no longer allowed to make mistakes and it is not a matter of physical perfection. It is something like: 'Let your behaviour be such that you can stand before God in all honesty.' But being at one with God sometimes also means that you must give up something; it costs you; it hurts! That aspect is found in circumcision.

Among the Arabs circumcision existed even before Muhammad: the new religion simply adopted the ritual. For that matter, there is not a single text to be found in the Qu'ran relating to circumcision, and in the writings of the exegetists one has to wait for two hundred years after the death of the Prophet, when El Bokhari (810–870), a Persian jurist and theologian, reports Muhammad as having said: 'Five acts make up our tradition: circumcision, the removal of the pubic hair, the depilation of the armpits and the clipping of the moustache and nails.' This is part of the *Sunna*, the book recording the acts and pronouncements of the prophet Muhammad and his followers. In fact circumcision is not compulsory for Muslims, but is a voluntary act following the example of the Prophet, amounting to a moral obligation, which means in practice that every male Muslim is circumcised. It is a rite of passage on the road to full membership of the religious community, with the associated rights and duties. This is probably the main reason why the circumcision is carried out only when the boy is slightly older, usually between the ages of two and twelve.

The Jewish author Philo of Alexandria (AD 25–50) was the first to put forward hygienic motives for circumcision. In hot dry climates sand, insects, larvae and suchlike are difficult to remove, and this may result in inflammation. The fear of paraphimosis also played a part. Paraphimosis may occur when in a mild form of phimosis the foreskin is retracted as far as the corona of the glans penis and cannot return. This causes the glans and the foreskin to swell through engorgement with blood and the formation of oedemas, resulting in pain and panic. Doctors talk of a 'Spanish collar', after the starched ruff collars worn by prominent Spaniards in the sixteenth and seventeenth centuries.

Paraphimosis can be resolved by squeezing the glans and the foreskin with the whole hand and with steadily increasing pressure carefully emptying the swollen tissue. If that does not work, the doctor can use the so-called Dundee technique: making multiple punctures with a fine needle and then suspending the swollen tip in a cup of sugar, so that the fluid from the tissue is quickly absorbed. This trick has been copied from vets, who use it on cows with swollen and prolapsed uteri, which have been through a protracted delivery and cannot be pushed back inside.

As described previously the glans is the end of the *corpus spongiosum*, the erectile tissue compartment surrounding the urethra. In erection the glans swells, but the internal pressure remains lower than that in the *corpora cavernosa*. The glans is lined with a sensitive mucous membrane and is normally sheathed with foreskin, which consists on the inside of mucous membrane and on the outside of skin. Since the vagina is also lined with mucous membrane, the penis can easily slide back and forth. Both the glans and the foreskin contain numerous fine nerve endings, which heighten sexual pleasure. This means that the foreskin is also an important sexual organ, the simple rubbing of which can lead to an ejaculation. If it is removed, a sexually significant part of the penis is lost, and continuous friction causes a layer of callus to form.

Any Jewish man may carry out a circumcision, but the ritual (*brit milah*) is mostly performed by the *mohel*. It is a religious obligation, and should normally take place on the eighth day after birth. General principles of treatment if there are medical problems are laid down in the Shulchan Aruch. Circumcision is, for instance, forbidden if there are

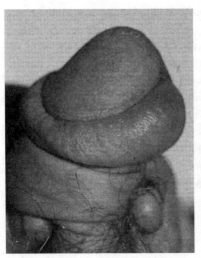
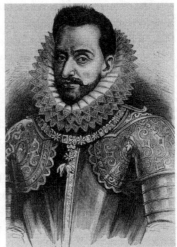

The 'Spanish collar'.

any indications for haemophilia; if in any family two sons have died or if two sisters of the mother have each lost a child from bleeding after circumcision, the following son must not be circumcised. This rule is regarded as the very first indication of haemophilia, a disease that we know today is inherited through the maternal line.

The *sandak*, a kind of godfather, holds the child on his lap during the ceremony. The *mohel* pulls the whole foreskin up to the glans and pushes the skin into the slot of a protective plate, after which the foreskin is cut along the line of the slot without anaesthetic. Formerly the wound was sucked clean orally by the *mohel* (*mezizah*), but when it was found that syphilis, tuberculosis and diphtheria (and nowadays AIDS too) could be passed on in this way, a suction instrument was introduced for the purpose. The wound used to be treated with *mohel* flour, a powder made of ground oakwood; nowadays it is bandaged. Incidentally, last century it was the custom among the Falaches, a Jewish sect in what was then Abyssinia, to circumcise even still-born male babies before they were put in their coffins, so that when they were resurrected they would be immediately recognized as Jews.

For both Jews and Muslims circumcision is surrounded by prayers and rituals. Among Indonesian Muslims circumcision is called *sunat*. Sometimes a *dukun* (village doctor) or *bong* (imman) performs the ceremony, but usually the procedure is carried out by a layman. In Java the foreskin is sometimes cut only lengthways: a flat piece of bamboo is pushed between the glans and the foreskin, after which the foreskin is severed. Because the glans is initially uncomfortably sensitive after circumcision, the boys are put under cold running water. To protect the glans from grazing they wear half a coconut shell over their penis which hangs from a string round their waist.

The television film *The Winds of War* showed how after the invasion of Poland in 1939 foreigners, including Americans, travelled back to Berlin through the German lines. Jews and people with Jewish-looking faces and Jewish names were singled out. In cases of doubt the Nazis looked to see whether the men were circumcised or not. In the film an American minister travelling with the group protested: 'All Americans are circumcised, me too.' Under the Nazi threat many foreskin-restorations were carried out in this period. In fact, these are age-old practices: as long ago as the second century BC there were Jewish apostates who were anxious to imitate the ways of their Hellenistic overlords and to participate in sporting events in the athletics school in Jerusalem.

In ancient Rome too there were Jews who because of sanctions against them wished to undo their circumcision. Obviously there were successful methods even at that time, since, when the law banning circumcision was repealed, the requirements that a circumcision had to meet were further tightened by the rabbis. The foreskin must be completely removed, so that no tissue remained for possible experiments.

Then there is the well-known discussion about King David's 'marble foreskin', since Michelangelo's celebrated statue of this Jewish patriarch shows him apparently uncircumcised. Scholars had a field day with this and finally declared that Michelangelo knew exactly what he was doing: King David lived around 1000 BC, and it was not until after 300 BC that the circumcision laws were tightened. Before that time only a small fringe of the foreskin was removed, which is exactly what one sees in Michelangelo's sculpture, where the foreskin does not completely cover the glans . . .

Religious circumcision confronts many surgeons, urologists or plastic surgeons with a dilemma. On the one hand there is the right to physical and intellectual integrity, and the individual's right to self-determination, and on the other there is freedom of religion. And religions sometimes have archaic rules. A recent Dutch government proved pro-active on this point and removed ritual circumcision from the standard health insurance package.

Health circumcision

In 1870 an American orthopaedic surgeon launched the notion that a whole range of ailments, rheumatism, asthma, kidney infections, bed-wetting, alcoholism, sterility and venereal disease, could be cured by circumcision. Sayre, the surgeon concerned, was acclaimed as the 'Columbus of the foreskin'.

At the beginning of the twentieth century an American magazine hypothesized that the low incidence of cervical cancer in Jewish women might be a result of Jewish men being circumcised. Although this hypothesis was not confirmed by scientific research, there was a massive overreaction: since then virtually all American male babies have been circumcised, mostly in hospital. In 1900 a quarter of male Americans had been circumcised. This so-called health circumcision, on medical grounds, was used in Europe in the Victorian period, but at that time to prevent masturbation.

When the army medical service published reports to the effect that uncircumcised soldiers were much more susceptible to venereal disease than their circumcised colleagues, circumcision was recommended as a preventative health measure. The result of this was that by the late 1960s some 90 per cent of the male population was circumcised. In 1969 there were the first stirrings of resistance, but it was not until

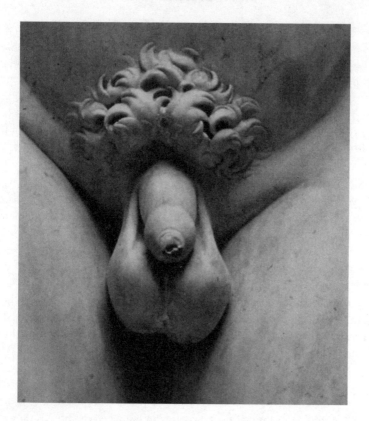

David's private
parts.

1990 that there was a real sea change in America. A lobby group for
circumcised men was set up and there were direct appeals to the media:
'We don't cut babies' ears off because they need washing behind them,
do we?' Members could not only commiserate with each other, but
could also swap experiences about all kinds of methods of restoring
the foreskin. These included obtaining 'new' tissue by careful stretching of the remains of the foreskin, involving the use of clamps, plasters
and elastic bands. Homosexuals, as so often with these kinds of problems, were the trailblazers. From San Anselmo in the United States the
anti-circumcision lobby distributes its newsletter *No-circ*, which reports
on successes achieved, like a ban on female circumcision, which is
regarded as a first step in the struggle against male circumcision. In a
statement the movement argues that doctors who perform a ritual
circumcision are infringing the ancient medical adage *primum non
nocere*, do not inflict harm. Even the UN charter on human rights is
invoked: no one shall be subjected to torture, or inhuman or humiliating treatment.

In early 2007, as a result of publications in the authoritative journal *The Lancet*, there were unexpected developments. A study in Kenya

headed by scientists from Johns Hopkins University (Baltimore) involved 2,784 HIV-negative men aged between eighteen and 24. The men were either circumcised or their circumcision had been postponed for two years. After two years 4.2 per cent of the second group had become infected with the HIV virus, whereas in the group of immediately circumcised men the percentage was 2.1!

In Uganda a comparable study was conducted by a team from the University of Illinois, only this time with 4,996 HIV-negative men between fifteen and 49. This study also showed a halving of the risk of HIV infection. The tenor of the various reactions was more or less unanimous: because of the enormous potential of circumcision, within Southern Africa alone a reduction of 3.7 million HIV infections and 2.7 million deaths from AIDS, the procedure had to be seen as a preventative measure. This marked a return to 'health circumcision'.

chapter eight

Voluntary and Involuntary Sterility

Forced sterilization

The controversial history of sterilization in men, vasectomy, begins with Cooper's publication of 1832 on the severing of the seminal duct in dogs. The first sterilization was carried out in the United States at the end of the nineteenth century in order to prevent the spread of crime. There was a fear that the USA would be inundated by mentally and socially inferior people. The procedure was also carried out in the United Kingdom, but in this case on eugenic grounds, to protect the race from self-destruction by its own descendants. At the beginning of the twentieth century Sharp reported on 450 sterilizations he had carried out in the state of Indiana on members of the Reformed Church. In their case vasectomy was intended to suppress masturbation. It was performed without anaesthetic and took no longer than three minutes. The severed end of the duct on the testicle side was left open so that the sperm cells could drain away freely and be absorbed by the body. In 1907 a law was introduced in Indiana that permitted the sterilization of 'mental defectives' and the 'insane and feeble-minded' for eugenic reasons. In the following decades similar laws were passed by 32 states, while twelve also legalized the forced sterilization of criminals. Up to 1960 over 60,000 sterilizations were carried out for the above-mentioned reasons.

In Germany in 1933 vasectomy was made to serve eugenics, based on 'modern racial hygiene'. In the first year after its introduction 28,000 sterilizations were carried out. In 1936 Adolf Hitler discussed sterilization with the German cardinal Faulhaber, the Archbishop of Munich. Hitler had argued for the sterilization of those with hereditary defects, and is reported as saying the following: 'The operation is simple and does not make the man unsuitable for an occupation or marriage, and now we are being thwarted by the church.' Cardinal Faulhaber is supposed to have said: 'Chancellor, the state is not being forbidden by the church to remove these harmful individuals from the community within the framework of the laws on public decency and given a genuine emergency. But instead of physical mutilation other methods must be tried, and such a means exists: the internment of people with hereditary defects.'

Internment camps amounted to concentration camps; such an institution fell within the laws on public decency and sterilization did not. Sterilization led to sexual pleasure without reproduction and that in the view of Catholic moral theologians could not possibly be permitted. For the ordinary Catholic sexual intercourse had repercussions, as Uta Ranke describes in her book *Eunuchs for the Kingdom of Heaven*.

In 1935 a question came from Aachen to the Holy See as to whether a forcibly sterilized man could be admitted to a church marriage. On 16 February the reply was received that the man's marriage must not be forbidden, since it involved an unjust coercive measure by the state.

In Sweden it has been possible since 1935, with the approval of a committee, to sterilize those whom 'the law has declared *non compos mentis*', or who because of a psychiatric condition are deemed unsuitable for parenthood. In 1948 a law was promulgated to control sterilization on eugenic grounds; in practice many sterilizations were actually performed for socio-economic reasons. Between 1948 and 1962 14,000 sterilizations were carried out in Japan, and the number of illegal sterilizations was estimated at four times that figure.

A large proportion of people with a mental handicap are not able to give informed consent with regard to sterilization. In those cases the carer should fulfil his/her obligations towards the parents or guardian and, with those who are of age, towards those charged with the person's welfare. If the handicapped person is capable of informed consent and is over the age of twelve but not yet sixteen, the permission of parent or guardian is also required. Everything seems perfectly regulated, but in practice the picture is different. When the parents of a strapping lad of fourteen with Down's syndrome asked me to have him sterilized, since their son had already made a spontaneous attempt at intercourse, I acceded to their request without hesitation. Some readers might think that a Down's syndrome male with his 47 chromosomes cannot father children, but in certain circumstances that is perfectly possible.

Even today forced sterilizations take place, and not only of the mentally handicapped. The following story may serve as an illustration: Patient A, a 37-year-old man of Iranian origin, came to the urology clinic after having failed for the third time to father a child. His ejaculate repeatedly contained almost no sperm cells. After some years' residence in the Netherlands both he and his wife wanted to extend their family. He had fled from Iran for political reasons, having endured extended periods of torture, including electric shocks to his genitalia, which had often rendered him unconscious. Echographic examination led to a diagnosis of an epididymal cyst on the right side and on the left; the head of the epididymis was irregular; the testicles themselves showed no abnormalities. At the patient's request the diagnostic process was continued in our clinic after two years, and it was decided to perform an exploratory operation under anaesthetic. When sections of tissue from the testes were examined the pathologist found a slight disruption of sperm production on both sides, though adult sperm cells were present. After the removal of scar tissue, non-soluble green knotted stitches were observed on both sides, consistent with a post-vasectomy condition. The loose ends were stitched back together on both sides, without any post-operative complications. When the hospital did a follow-up check, the patient indicated that he had absolutely no knowledge of the sterilization.

Sometimes men are ignorant of the fact that they have undergone sterilization. Another illustrative case history: A 47-year-old man was referred to me by a gynaecologist in relation to the patient's involuntary childlessness with his new partner. He had two children from a previous marriage. Three examinations by the gynaecologist showed a complete absence of sperm cells. In another hospital a section of testicular tissue had been removed under local anaesthetic. The production of sperm cells, spermatogenesis, was shown to be only slightly disrupted, which suggested an obstruction, for instance a double epididymal inflammation. When asked if he had had diseases or operations in the past, the patient's answer was negative. It was decided to explore further under anaesthetic. No obvious abnormalities were apparent to the touch, but after incision it soon became clear that he had been sterilized: the gap between the two ends of the seminal duct was so small on both sides that it had not been felt and likewise on inspection of his shaved scrotum the tiny scars were virtually invisible. The ducts were rejoined on both sides, and there were no post-operative complications. At a follow-up check the patient mentioned that in the years before and following his divorce his alcohol intake had been very high, and that he could remember little or nothing from that time. When asked about the case the referring gynaecologist said that he had information only from the GP of the present partner. Three months after the restorative operation microscopic examination showed over 20 million spermatozoa per millilitre, and it was soon possible to fulfil the desire for children.

When divorced people enter into a new relationship, there is of course a good chance that they will not have the same GP. If the referral process in relation to an unfulfilled desire for children subsequently begins with the woman, usually only her medical records are forwarded. In this case the urologist had omitted to request possibly relevant information on the man from the GP.

The World Health Organization

In the 1970s a large-scale programme was launched by the World Health Organization in India and elsewhere to combat over-population, in which millions of men were sterilized. The same happened in China under government pressure. For some decades Chinese doctors had already been using alternatives to vasectomy, including a technique requiring only three instruments (an important factor in developing countries), the so called 'no-scalpel' technique, that is, no scalpel but a sharp clip, a pair of scissors and another clip for fixation of the seminal ducts.

The Chinese doctors claimed that with the aid of this technique haemorrhaging was less frequent than in conventional vasectomies, an important factor in a country where at the time sterilization of men was more or less obligatory after the birth of the first child, and in addition was less time-consuming. Another Chinese technique was based on quickly pricking the outer surface of the seminal duct, after which a blunt-ended needle was inserted in the duct on both sides. On one side a blue dye (methylene blue) was injected and on the other a red one (Congo red). If after the procedure the man's urine was red, the operation had most probably been a success! When the needles appeared to be properly in position on both sides, a caustic fluid was injected, causing a build-up of scar tissue which blocked the seminal ducts. Initially phenol was used, and later carbolic acid with cyanoacrylate. The advantage of this method of sterilization was the speed with which it could be performed. In any case the procedure was irreversible. To this end the Chinese had started using polyurethane and later silicones, but the use of polyurethane in the seminal duct was not initially permitted by the WHO since there was a chance it might be carcinogenic. The use of silicones, however, was sanctioned by the WHO at the end of the 1980s, in the first instance for plugging the Fallopian tubes via the vagina and the uterus. When asked, the Chinese were not able to give the exact composition of their silicones, so a Dutch company and Dutch urologists were called in. A joint workshop was held, which was also attended by Indonesian urologists. Chinese men from an area in the province of Shandong were used as test subjects. This method was of great interest to the Indonesians, since many Muslims have religious objections to conventional sterilization. Basically their religion forbids

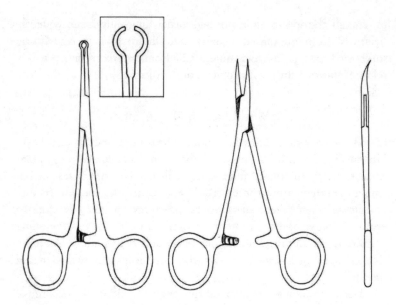

Chinese instruments for use in vasectomy.

the violation of the body, and any contraceptive procedure should be reversible. The Dutch doctors were of course focused on a potentially easily reversible form of sterilization: removing a plug is much easier than a lengthy, expensive operation in which the ends have to be sewn back together.

At the workshop it soon became clear that the Chinese had not succeeded in achieving sterility in 100 per cent of the men treated with plugs, an outcome which would never be acceptable in Western culture in countries where sterilization was on a completely voluntary basis. Failed sterilizations have sometimes led to (successful) claims for damages, though this virtually never happens today, since every doctor performing an operation will inform the patient about the impossibility of guaranteeing absolute sterility. Carrying out a vasectomy entails an obligation to perform to the best of one's abilities, not an obligation to guarantee a certain result: an important legal distinction.

The type of vasectomy which involves the removal of a section of seminal duct is at present considered one of the most practical ways of achieving sterility. With Nepal, the Netherlands, Yemen, Bulgaria and India, the United Kingdom is among the few countries in the world where more men than women have been sterilized. Countries where vasectomy is considered completely unacceptable include the Dominican Republic, El Salvador, Honduras, Jamaica and Tunisia. What kind of people opt for vasectomy? Mainly men over 30, with a high educational level, an above-average income and a complete family. Many of them feel that it is now 'their turn' to contribute to contraception.

Though the operation may be regarded as simple by some, the great variety of techniques used suggests a different picture. The great majority of surgeons use local anaesthetic, beginning with the nerves in the seminal cord. In the 1960s it was not unusual for a man to go straight back to work after the procedure, but today patients are recommended to take things easy, at least on the day itself. An experienced doctor can perform the procedure in less than fifteen minutes, though it is sometimes difficult to locate the seminal duct, particularly if the scrotum is rather compact. Matters are complicated if the man involved disregards advice and arrives by bike in winter. For reasons of temperature regulation the layer of muscle beneath the skin of the scrotum is tautened, making it more difficult for the urologist to take hold of the seminal duct.

Bearing in mind the possibility that the procedure may one day have to be reversed, it is sensible to carry out the vasectomy high in the scrotum. To check whether the operation has been successful, the ejaculate is examined under the microscope after three months for the presence of spermatozoa (there is no point in doing this any sooner). In those three months it is advisable to ejaculate as often as possible: after vasectomy the patient is not immediately sterile, since downstream from the point of ligature spermatozoa are still making their way towards the outside world. The criterion for sterility is the absence of sperm cells; according to urological guidelines it is sufficient if after three months there are only a few cells visible, provided that these are immobile. On problem is that if a patient submits ejaculate that has spent some time out of the body, the spermatozoa will invariably have failed to survive. One thing is certain: if after a vasectomy living sperm cells remain visible, alarm bells should start sounding. In 2004 the US Food and Drug Administration (FDA) approved a new vasectomy

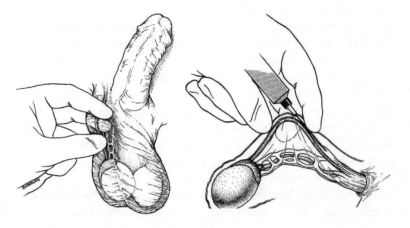

Presentation of seminal duct and local anaesthetic.

technique, in which the seminal ducts are not severed or cauterized but are closed off with the aid of a special clip, Vasclip. The technique is designed to make a restorative operation easier, but has not yet been approved in Europe.

Spontaneous recanalization

From the very beginning the occurrence of spontaneous recanalization, the growing together of the severed ends of the seminal ducts, has been one of the main problems associated with vasectomy. As long ago as the 1950s it became clear that if one simply tied off the seminal duct there was virtually always recanalization, and even after severing in several places there was also spontaneous recanalization. If a length of 3 cm was removed, but the sheath of the duct remained intact, the same thing happened. Recanalization did not occur if the sheath was also removed.

Recanalization is still a problem, and is found in between 1 in 1,000 and 1 in 2,000 men who have 'had themselves fixed'. The risk is higher if after the vasectomy a spermagranuloma develops. A granuloma is created by leakage of spermatozoa on the testicle side, despite effective ligature of the end of the seminal duct. Tying off is actually not all that easy, since the seminal duct has a thick wall of muscle, so that there is a risk that the stitch will be pulled too tight and will sever the duct. Partly for this reason many urologists decide for reasons of safety to cauterize the tied-off ends. It is also a good idea to sew a section of different tissue between the two ends, preventing them from coming into contact.

The complications of vasectomy are quite often underestimated. Whichever way you look at it, vasectomy is an odd procedure; if a surgeon were to remove a section of intestine and close off both ends, he or she would be immediately committed to a lunatic asylum, if necessary by force . . .

From puberty to death millions of sperm cells pass along these tubes that resemble liquorice shoelaces. After vasectomy the 'little creatures' can no longer do this. Upstream of the blockage all is woe and affliction, with dead and dying spermatozoa, and of course that can lead to ailments: a painfully swollen epididymis, pain in ejaculating, the previously mentioned spermagranuloma and tears in the wall of the extremely long tube which the epididymis in fact is. Sperm cells may leak through those tears, causing inflammation and antibody formation, since spermatozoa are regarded as basically alien, having only half the normal number of chromosomes.

In the past few decades surgeons and urologists have perhaps made things a little too easy for themselves in failing to dispense complete information on the possible downside of vasectomy. Many men would be deterred if they were told that approximately 5 per cent of sterilized men have chronic testicular pain. Men who already suffer from testicular pain should certainly not have themselves sterilized. Other reasons not to be sterilized include childlessness, a serious or chronic illness in one's partner and the lack of a permanent relationship. In addition anyone contemplating the procedure should be warned of continued bleeding and/or haemorrhaging (10% to 20% chance) and infection (2% to 10% chance).

Restorative operations

In 1888 Bernhard Bardenheuer (1839–1913), a German surgeon who specialized in genito-urinary surgery, was the first to try to connect the seminal duct and the testicle in a man whose epipidymis had been removed because of tuberculosis, and in 1934 a thorough survey of all attempts made up to then was published by the German researcher F. Spath. Spath himself experimented on dogs: at the point where he had sewn together the two ends he left behind a soluble sewing thread made of catgut, thus preventing premature blockage by scar tissue. His results were disappointing, especially when the ends were tied together under tension. Vaso-vasostomy – the name by which a restorative operation after vasectomy is known – fell into obscurity. A few American researchers, however, persisted stubbornly into the 1960s and 1970s. Dogs proved to be excellent guinea-pigs. So what were the underlying difficulties related to a restorative operation? In the first place the spot where the ends were attached must not leak, or there would be an inflammatory reaction. It also became clear that the thread must not be under tension. Too large a section of the seminal duct must not be removed in sterilization and the ends must not contain too much scar tissue. Another finding was that tension could be produced by the simple fact that dogs, like humans, have hanging testicles.

In operating on humans use is often made of a splint, which is positioned outside the scrotum and removed after a few days. Stitching over a splint makes it impossible to sew up everything tightly. Initially many of those carrying out the operation removed a small section of testicle before finally deciding on a restorative operation. Later this was no longer considered necessary, at least if the testicles felt normal on physical examination. It also became clear that over half the men who had had a vasectomy had developed antibodies against their own sperm. However, a high level of antibodies does not mean that a restorative operation has no chance of success.

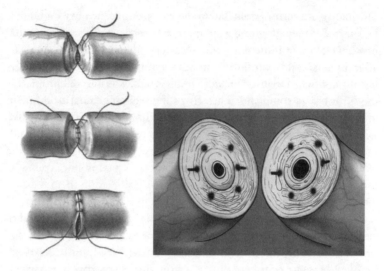

Vaso-vasostomy.

About 90,000 vasectomies are carried out in the UK each year. Nearly 600 vasectomy reversals are done every year in NHS hospitals, but many more are performed privately. So, the exact number of vaso-vasostomies is not known. (In the Netherlands 2.5% of vasectomized males have reversal surgery.)

There is an 80 per cent chance of achieving adequate throughput in the seminal duct if the restorative operation takes place within ten years of sterilization. The longer the interval, the less chance of success. Incidentally, adequate throughput does not mean that it will be easy for the partner to become pregnant, since sperm quality is virtually always inferior to that of non-sterilized men, meaning that in many cases assisted reproductive methods are required. The number of men who regret undergoing a vasectomy is large, given the previously mentioned testicular pain. The chance that a patient will regret the decision increases the younger the age at which the vasectomy takes place. In men below 25 the chance is over 11 per cent.

The reader may think: 'Is anybody really sterilized at that age?' Well, not in 2007, but they were in the 1970s. In those days it was quite normal for young guys to have themselves sterilized. It was an age of doom and gloom, mainly fuelled by the alarming economic and social reports of the Club of Rome, which invoked the approaching apocalypse with almost Calvinist fervour.

Deterioration in sperm quality

In the early 1990s researchers at the University of Copenhagen analysed the scientific literature that had appeared between 1938 and 1991 on the quality of sperm, which had involved 15,000 men. They found that in 1940 the average number of spermatozoa per millilitre of seminal fluid was 116 million. By 1990 that had fallen to 66 million. The amount of semen (sperm cells and seminal fluid) produced per ejaculation had also fallen. The average for 1940 was 3.4 millilitres, for 1990 only 2.75 millilitres. These two findings pointed to a decline in male fertility. The researchers assumed that exposure to toxins like dioxins, alkylphenols, PCB and DDT played a significant part in this.

The standards for 'normal' sperm have been adjusted over the course of time: nowadays 20 million sperm cells per millilitre counts as the lower limit. If there is to be a chance of fertilization there must be a minimum of 5 million spermatozoa present in each millilitre of seminal fluid, but a minimum of 10 million is desirable and as was said in 2007, a minimum of 20 million was regarded as normal.

Spermatozoa are incredibly small: from the head to the tip of the tail they measure 0.05 mm with a maximum diameter of 0.0025 mm. The sperm cells of men, horses and zebras resemble each other, having the same shape of head and a long tail. They share these characteristics with the lancelet fish, the escargot and the water flea. A rat's sperm cells have a sickle-shaped head, while the hermit crab has beetle-like, exploding spermatozoa. If any of them touches an egg it leaps up and launches its genetic cargo into the interior of the egg.

The human male tadpole really is a miracle of design. It consists of three parts: the oval head, in which the genetic material is transported, an oblong thickened central section housing the engine room, and a tail which enables the sperm cell to steer towards the ovum. The fuel is sugar, which in the engine room is converted into adenosine phosphate. Very many spermatozoa die in the extremely acid vagina, and 40 per cent of the survivors are rejected at the entrance to the womb. Then half of the survivors swim into the wrong Fallopian tube, until finally one victor emerges in the sperm competition. Arriving at the ovum the chosen spermatozoon sheds its cap, or acrosome, which contains a special protein, releasing enzymes that enable the sperm cell to penetrate the ovum. So while a large number of sperm cells are required to make fertilization possible, quantity alone is not decisive: quality is also of great importance. This includes having a normal head and being able to swim fast in one direction, not swimming circuits but a long-distance race. If little of the sperm is up to standard, doctors speak of *oligo-terato-asthenospermia*. 'Oligo' indicates an insufficient quantity, 'terato' an excessive number of abnormal heads and 'astheno' poor mobility. If no spermatozoa are found in the ejaculate, it is called *azoospermia*.

Diagnostic methods in reduced male fertility

According to the WHO one can speak of reduced fertility where no conception has occurred after one year of frequent and unprotected intercourse. It is not completely clear what is meant by frequent. Eels mate once in their lives, taking a long time to become sexually mature. Many of these fish are over eighteen years old when they have sex for the first and last time somewhere in the shadowy depths of the Bermuda Triangle. After depositing their sperm or eggs, they die.

Although the vast majority of human couples see their wish for pregnancy fulfilled within a year, there remains a group with reduced fertility. The majority will eventually achieve a spontaneous pregnancy and a small percentage will remain involuntarily childless. The cause of reduced fertility may lie with the woman, the man or both simultaneously. A large WHO study showed that in 39 per cent of cases the cause of involuntary childlessness lay with the woman, in 20 per cent with the man and in 26 per cent with both partners. In 15 per cent no cause can be found.

Systematic and standardized examination of a woman with reduced fertility is carried out by a gynaecologist, and in the case of men by a urologist with a particular interest in this problem, who in most European countries is called an andrologist. Causes of reduced fertility include: inability to achieve an erection or a sufficiently hard erection, inability to ejaculate, a varicose vein, an obstruction due to sterilization or inflammation of the epididymis, absence of seminal ducts, hormonal problems, certain medications, undescended testicles and inflammation of the prostate. In many cases the cause unfortunately remains unknown.

There is no better characterization of reproductive problems than that given by the biologist Midas Dekkers:

> First you have to negotiate with some woman. You have to introduce yourself, say what you earn, what your father does . . .
> you can't buy an ovum anywhere. There's a whole tea cosy
> built around an ovum and the tea cosy doesn't want me to go
> anywhere near her ovum with my sperm. So I have to negotiate with her, dance with her, maybe even take dance classes . . .
> if that goes well and you're allowed to get to grips with her,
> there are millions of sperm at the start line ready for the off.
> Then we find that we as men should be ashamed of ourselves,
> since of all those sperm not one usually reaches its destination.
> The sperm we produce is totally shit sperm.

Investigation to determine the cause of male subfertility ('shit sperm') begins with questions about sexual development, illnesses, use of medication, smoking habits and external factors such as contact with toxic substances or frequent and protracted exposure to high temperatures. In addition attention will be paid to family illnesses and genetic disorders in the man or his partner. Various diseases are associated with fertility problems and if an unfulfilled desire for children is successfully treated they may be transmitted. Olfactory disorders and abnormalities in vision may be associated with a defect in the pineal gland (hypophysis). A number of genetic diseases are associated with a typical physical build, which will be immediately recognized by an experienced doctor. The patient will also be asked about certain personal habits: thermal underwear, use of saunas, intensive practising of sport, excessive alcohol use – all examples which may adversely affect fertility. The physical examination begins with looking at possible signs of breast formation, the pattern of hair growth and the measuring of height and weight. The examination of the groin area, penis, testicles, epididymides, seminal ducts and prostate is the counterpart of the gynaecological examination. There will also be a check for any variocele, which must be carried out with the man in standing position. Additional examination includes repeated examination of sperm – abnormalities found on one occasion need not be significant, since that could caused even by a flu bug – and hormone tests.

Closer examination

In the microscopic examination of sperm one looks, for example, at the number of sperm cells, their mobility and their shape. The volume of the sperm sample and the degree of acidity are also recorded. It is important that there should have been no ejaculation for three days: research has shown that that is when sperm quality is at its highest, and in addition different sperm samples can in that way be compared over time. We find that it is difficult for many men to produce sperm in the laboratory. However, if the sperm sample is obtained in more familiar surroundings, it is important that the sperm is delivered to the laboratory within the hour. The sperm must be collected directly into a jar provided for the purpose – the use of a patient's own jars is not to be recommended. The same applies to catching the sperm in a condom: rubber and latex are harmful to sperm cells. Of course it is crucial that *all* the sperm ejaculated is collected. If something gets lost, there is no point in taking the rest of the sperm to the laboratory. It is much better to arrange a new date with the lab.

Echography is a painless form of examination using sound waves, with which organs and blood vessels can be examined. Echography in the case of a subfertile man concerns mainly the contents of the scrotum, the groin, the prostate and the seminal glands. An echo can give indications of abnormalities in the testicle (inflammation, tumours), the epididymsis (engorgement, inflammation) and in the membranes surrounding the testicle (hydrocele). In combination with a measurement of the flow speed (colour Doppler echography), examination of the seminal cord can help locate a varicose vein quickly. Echography of the prostate and seminal glands is called for if there is a suspicion of inflammation or if the volume of sperm is repeatedly too low. This examination is performed by the rectal insertion of an echo sensor, which is placed against the prostate. This is not painful and can be carried out in an outpatient department. In this way abnormalities of the prostate (inflammation, calcification, enlargement, cancer) and the seminal glands (engorgement, or absence) can be brought to light.

The level of hormones like LH, FSH, inhibine and testosterone in the blood can be measured. With the passage of time there is a clear reduction in inhibine concentration and an increase in FSH. Both phenomena point to reduced sperm production. This loss begins shortly after the age of 21. This is not, though, the first sign of aging: that has to be the loss of one's milk teeth.

Heredity

In about 20 per cent of men with fewer than 20 million sperm cells per millimetre a genetic abnormality is found. A genetic investigation is called for if during a physical examination abnormalities are found which might be consonant with a genetic disorder (for example, the absence of seminal ducts or certain genetic disorders occurring in the family). Investigation of genetic abnormalities in subfertile men has only taken off in the last few decades, partly as a result of new reproduction techniques. Genetic investigation consists of two parts: karyotyping and DNA examination. In karyotyping, all the chromosomes in a cell, generally a blood cell, are coloured and counted under the microscope and subsequently examined separately. The main abnormalities that may be found are: an abnormal number of chromosomes (46 is the norm) or an abnormality in one or more chromosomes, like the lack of a section of chromosome. The section may have transferred to another chromosome (translocation) or been lost (deletion). Klinefelter's syndrome is the best-known example of an abnormal number. At least 1 in every 1,000 newborn boys have this syndrome. In the great majority of cases these men are infertile.

One of the most striking phenomena in Klinefelter's syndrome is the marked underdevelopment of the testicles, which usually do not grow beyond the size of a pea. Other characteristics are a relatively short penis, the formation of mammary glands, greater than average height, sparse beard growth and little pubic hair, which in addition often has a female growth pattern, namely with a horizontal upper limit. A man with an extra x chromosome is bound to be effeminate, would seem to be the obvious assumption, but that is totally wrong. And it is equally wrong to imagine that such a man is necessarily bisexual. If boys with Klinefelter's syndrome receive testosterone treatment in puberty, they grow into very masculine men, quite able to hold their own sexually!

DNA diagnosis

In recent years DNA diagnosis has become a rapidly developing field: more and more syndromes are being shown to be genetically determined and in a number of diseases it has become clear that a small part of the chromosome, the gene, is not functioning properly. An example of this is cystic fibrosis, a genetic disorder affecting a gene of chromosome number seven. This poorly functioning gene causes thick sticky mucus in, for example, the airways and the pituitary gland. Blockages of these organs lead to chronic airway infections and growth problems. In many cases the epididymides, the seminal duct and the seminal glands are affected by this ailment. Because sperms are actually being produced in the testicles it is sometimes possible for a sufferer of cystic fibrosis and his partner to achieve a pregnancy through ICSI, though a child fathered in this way risks developing a form of cystic fibrosis. For this reason examination of the man and if necessary of the woman is necessary prior to such treatment.

Recently the gene important in sperm production, the AZF gene, was found in the male chromosome. Minor writing errors in the order of the DNA molecules lead to disruptions in sperm cell production. Mutations in the AZF gene are found in between 5 and 15 per cent of all men with poor sperm quality. In the event of successful assisted reproduction these will be passed on to male descendants. This is yet another reason in cases of very poor sperm quality to consult a clinical geneticist.

Azoospermia and Sertoli cell only

When investigating infertility one regularly encounters azoospermia, the condition where no sperm cells at all are present in the ejaculate.

The number of new cases per year in the Netherlands is estimated at 300 to 400, of which two-thirds are caused by abnormalities in the production of sperm cells and about a third by a 'kink' in the duct system, or an obstruction.

The firm diagnosis of 'obstructive azoospermia' is made by microscopic examination of a section the size of a grain of rice from the larger of the two testicles. A Johnsen score is given, which is obtained by assessing the sperm-cell forming tubules for the degree of maturation from stem cell to 'mature' sperm cells. The presence of fully grown sperm cells gives a score of ten, nine or eight, the presence of spermatids, sperm cells that are not quite mature, gives a score of seven or six, spermatocytes five or four and only spermatogonia, sperm cells that are far from mature, a score of three. The Johnsen score has a strong correlation with the quality of the spermatogenesis. With a normal spermatogenesis the average score is 9.4.

The Sertoli cell-only syndrome is one of the commonest causes of non-obstructive azoospermia. 'Sertoli cell-only' refers to what the pathologists see on microscopic examination of a section of testicular tissue, that is sperm-cell forming tubules that are too small, have a thickened wall and are coated only with Sertoli cells. No germinating sperm cells are found, let alone fully mature ones. Patients with Sertoli cell-only have a normal male body, but often rather small testicles. With them the level of FSH, the hormone that from the hypophysis prompts the testicles to produce sperm cells, is too high. The cause of the syndrome is unknown. Very exceptionally in the testicular biopsy small areas of normal sperm cell production are found alongside the Sertoli cell-only picture.

Nowadays sperm cells can be obtained directly from the testicle or the epididymis, so that no spermatozoa need be present in the ejaculate. Because of these new options it is necessary for the pathologist to make a careful distinction between a 'complete' and an 'incomplete' Sertoli cell-only syndrome. For this reason several biopsies are done in different directions. In Belgium by doing several 'open' testicular biopsies doctors succeeded in obtaining sperm cells from a third of these patients, which means that even with a serious disruption of sperm cell production, ICSI (see below) is sometimes possible.

Defying Darwin

The oldest form of assisted reproduction is artificial insemination, in which a syringe or a pipette is used to bring the sperm into close proximity with the mouth of the womb. In 1780 the Italian scientist Spallanzini was the first to do this successfully, with a bitch. In 1799

John Hunter was the first to carry out the procedure with a woman. The sperm involved was that of a man with a deformation of the urethra, and Hunter injected it into the vagina of the man's wife. The technique did not catch on: there was quite simply no one to be found who wanted to take on this 'blasphemous' process. It was 1866 before the American gynaecologist J. Marion Sims, later a celebrated figure, took up artificial insemination again, putting sperm directly into the womb. From that time on the treatment was used very sparingly, mostly with married couples where the husband had become infertile because of bilateral gonorrhaeal inflammation of the epididymis.

In his book *Fertility in Marriage and Ways of Influencing It*, Th. H. van de Velde gives an account of how the pioneering American researcher Robert Latou Dickinson (1861–1950) conveyed the sperm directly to the Fallopian tube via the womb. H. Sellheim constructed an apparatus, the *Tubenbesamer*, with which the sperm could be blown into the Fallopian tubes; G. Fraenkel went even further: his advice was that if for any reason the abdomen had to be opened up, the ejaculate or *punctuate* from the epididymis should be brought into the immediate vicinity of the ovaries . . . Yet another gynaecologist suggested the idea of injecting sperm directly into the abdominal cavity from the back of the vagina, reasoning that by no means all sperm cells would immediately perish and that a few might even reach one of the ovaries.

Today artificial insemination is practised mainly by farmers. Approximately 90 per cent of cows and between 10 and 30 per cent of pigs are artificially inseminated. From the point of view of the breeder artificial insemination has many advantages over natural servicing, including the non-transmission of sexually transferable diseases.

Up to the mid-1970s artificial insemination was the only method of assisted reproduction available to help those suffering from involuntary childlessness. However, in the 1970s researchers and doctors developed a totally new kind of assisted fertilization: in-vitro fertilization (IVF). Two countries played a pioneering role – Australia and Great Britain – and four men are regarded as *the* founding fathers: the Britons Patrick Steptoe and Robert Edwards and the Australians Alan Trounson and Carl Wood.

Ultimately it was the British pair who took the crown: in 1978 Steptoe and Edwards were able to present the first 'test-tube baby' to the world. The miracle baby's name was Louise Brown. Incidentally, her sister Natalie, four years younger, was to be the first woman conceived by IVF herself to become a mother, only this time in the natural way. ICSI is a complementary technique developed by Dr Gianpiero Palermo at the Free University of Brussels. In ICSI a single living sperm cell is introduced into the ovum with a micropipette. The first experiments were carried out on mice, and in 1991 the first pregnancy was induced in a woman using ICSI. By 2005 more than 400,000 had been born through ICSI worldwide.

As of 2007 in Western Europe it is estimated that one in forty children were born with the help of the test tube – over one million babies worldwide – and if one includes other fertility-enhancing treatments, the proportion rises to one in twenty: these figures are hard to dismiss. Women not eligible for test-tube fertilization are those who are obese, those over the age of forty and those with 'bad' ovaries. The last condition can be tested by determining the level of FSH in the blood. Assisted fertilization methods include IUI, ICSI, PESA, TESE, TESA. The table below gives an overview.

Treatment		What exactly is it?
IUI	Intrauterine insemination	The injecting of sperm cells into the uterus
IVF	In-vitro fertilization	Fertilization in the test tube
ICSI	Intracytoplasmatic sperm injection	Injecting a sperm cell into an ovum
PESA	Percutaneous epididymal sperm aspiration	Aspiration via the skin of sperm cells from the epididymis
TESE	Testicular sperm extraction	Obtaining sperm cells from testicular tissue

One of the biggest problems in assisted reproduction techniques is the occurrence of multiple pregnancies. The risk of course increases in proportion to the number of embryos replaced. With multiple births delivery carries higher risks and there are frequent premature births, meaning that the babies not only spend a long period in hospital but also run the risk of, for example, retarded development. Doctors usually aim to replace as few embryos as possible.

Intracytoplasmatic sperm injection (ICSI) is nothing more than a complement to in-vitro fertilization (IVF). In ICSI a single living sperm cell is introduced into the ovum with a micropipette. Through the microscope the analyst selects a suitably mobile sperm cell, gives it a tap on the tail so that it is stunned for a second, then picks it up with a pipette and injects it into the ovum. As a potential parent you naturally hope that a Rolls Royce sperm cell is picked up, but the fact remains that you are defying Charles Darwin . . . In ICSI at least, processes that play a part in natural fertilization are bypassed. In con-

ICSI.

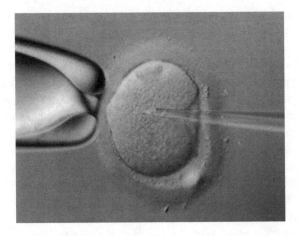

trast to IVF, ICSI requires only one mobile sperm cell per ovum. In cases of azoospermia through obstruction, PESA is the most common technique: with obstruction the number of properly mobile sperm cells is highest in the head of the epididymis, with a production problem the chance of finding mobile sperm cells is greatest in the tail.

In PESA a needle is inserted into the epididymis under local anaesthetic and withdrawn as suction continues. The needle is connected to a syringe via a tube, which is then injected with growing medium so that the content can be assessed by an analyst for the number of mobile sperm cells. This procedure can be repeated several times in a session. Usually one starts on the side of the larger testicle, and if the count is low one can try the other side.

In a TESE treatment sperm cells are taken from the testicle itself, and subsequently sperm cells are extracted in a laboratory from the section of testicular tissue removed. This has the advantage that a section of testicular tissue can immediately be obtained for the Johnsen score.

The treatment of fertility problems is generally felt to be very onerous. There are many stressful events, including (for women) daily hormone injections, blood samples, and diagnostic procedures such as exploratory operations, and masturbating to order and 'epididymal sperm aspiration' in men. Intercourse tends to become reproduction-led, potentially placing the desire for sex under pressure. In addition there is the situation of being constantly tossed back and forth between hope and fear. It becomes particularly burdensome when one wants to keep treatments secret from family, friends and colleagues. Taking time off work without letting colleagues in on the secret necessarily involves some fibbing.

Freezing sperm cells

Freezing sperm cells, cryopreservation, is important mainly to young men with testicular cancer who after removal of the affected testicle face a course of chemotherapy. Occasionally a man presents for sterilization, while expressing the wish that his sperm be stored in advance of the procedure. Such a wish cannot be met with the normal health service, though he can have sperm frozen by commercial institutions. Anyone thinking that sperm banks are a twentieth-century human invention is wrong: for several million years the male springtail has been consistently distributing scores of sperm droplets in the form of a chain. When the female insect's eggs are mature, she goes to the sperm depot and takes one.

Simple freezing of sperm cells leads to shrinkage of the cell, loss of fluid and sometimes cracks, resulting in loss of function. There was a great step forward after the discovery of glycerol, which could counter the above processes. In freezing for cryopreservation liquid nitrogen is used, cooled to –196 degrees Celsius. One sperm sample can be used to fill between five and fifteen ampoules containing 0.3 millilitres. Depending on the situation between one and three batches of sperm will be frozen. After freezing, one ampoule is defrosted in order to assess the mobility of the spermatozoa: the percentage of mobile sperm that continues to move after freezing or defrosting respectively varies from 5 to 50 per cent. With a concentration of mobile sperm of at least one million per millilitre in the initial sample, there is a reasonable chance of mobile sperm after the defrosting of the whole amount. This is important information when ICSI is being considered, since only mobile sperm can be used.

The ampoules of frozen sperm are distributed across two vats in order to reduce the chance of loss as far as possible. It is impossible to assign every individual a deep-freeze vat of their own, so that the sperm of several men is stored in a single deep-freeze vat. Occasionally tiny cracks in the ampoules appear during freezing, so that the contents may come into contact with the liquid nitrogen. In this way viruses and microbes can in theory be released and come into contact with the frozen seed of other men. Because of this risk the man is required by law to be tested in advance for infectious diseases such as AIDS and hepatitis.

Sperm donorship

The first recorded sperm donation that took place in a medical center was carried out with few of the ethical considerations that are mandated in clinics today: it was performed in 1884 at Philadelphia medical school for an infertile couple. Instead of taking the sperm from the husband, the doctor chloroformed the woman, then let his medical students vote which of them was the 'best looking', with that elected one providing the sperm for the insemination. After talking to the husband, they decided it was best not to let the woman know.

Sperm donation can be a morally contentious issue. Couples in heterosexual relationships considering sperm donation as a solution to childlessness may view it as preserving the sexual integrity of their relationship. However, sperm donation does not maintain the reproductive integrity of a relationship in that the woman's sexual partner is not the biological father of her child, and it is the sperm donor, not the partner, who has reproduced himself.

However, others point out that the process is essentially a sexual one: a woman's innate sexuality may be the reason why a child is wanted, the donor has to be screened for sexually transmitted diseases which could be passed on through the use of his sperm, and the donor has to sexually stimulate himself in order to produce the sperm samples which are used for achieving pregnancies in women to whom he is not related. Some would argue that it is impossible to distinguish sexuality from reproduction, and that the reason for preserving sexual integrity is to preserve reproductive integrity.

The use of sperm donation is increasingly popular among unmarried women and single or coupled lesbians. Indeed, some sperm banks and fertility clinics, particularly in the US, Denmark and the UK have a predominance of women being treated with donor sperm who fall within these groups and their publicity is aimed at them. This produces many ethical issues around the ideals of conventional parenting and has wider issues for society as a whole, including the issues of the role of men as parents, the issue of family support for children, and the issue of financial support for women with children.

Some donor children grow up wishing to find out who their fathers were, but others may be wary of embarking on such a search since they fear they may find scores of half-siblings who have been produced from the same sperm donor. Even though local laws or rules may restrict the numbers of offspring from a single donor, there are no worldwide limitations or controls and most sperm banks will 'onsell' and export all their remaining stocks of vials of sperm when local maxima have been attained.

However, others would argue that sperm donation has liberated the way in which women can control their reproductive lives and that it has enabled many men as sperm donors to father children which they would not want or wish to support but which they know will fulfil a desperate biological and social need for the women who bear them.

Many donees do not tell the child that they were conceived as a result of sperm donation, or, when non-anonymous donor sperm has been used, they do not tell the child until it is old enough for the clinic to provide the contact information about the donor.

For children who find out after a long period of secrecy, their main grief is usually not the fact that they are not the genetic child of the couple who have raised them, but the fact that the parent or parents have kept information from them or lied to them, causing loss of trust. Furthermore, the overturning of their knowledge of who their parents are may cause a lasting sense of imbalance and loss of control.

However, there are certain circumstances where the child very likely should be told: when many relatives know about the insemination, so that the child might find it out from somebody else; when the husband carries a significant genetic disease, relieving the child from fear of being a carrier; or where the child is found to suffer from a genetically transmitted disorder and it is necessary to take legal action which then identifies the donor.

Anonymous sperm donation is where the child and/or receiving couple will never get to know the identity of the donor, and non-anonymous when they will. A donor who makes a non-anonymous sperm donation is termed a known donor, open-identity or identity-release donor. Non-anonymous sperm donors are, to a substantially higher degree, driven by altruistic motives for their donations.

In any case, some information about the donor may be released to the woman/couple at the time of treatment. A limited donor information at most includes height, weight, eye, skin and hair colour. In Sweden, this is all the information a receiver gets. In the US, on the other hand, additional information may be given, such as a comprehensive biography and sound/video samples.

For most sperm recipients, anonymity of the donor is not of major importance at the obtainment or tryer-stage. The main reason for anonymity is that recipients think it would be easiest if the donor was completely out of the picture. However, some recipients regret not having chosen a non-anonymous donor years later, for instance when the child desperately wants to know more about the donor anyway.

There is a risk of bias in the information given by clinics or sperm banks regarding anonymity, making anonymous sperm donation seem more favourable than it may actually be, resulting from the fact that anonymous sperm donations are easier for the clinic or sperm bank to handle in the long term, because anonymity doesn't make them responsible for safely storing donor information for a long period of time. In addition, a majority of donors are anonymous, causing a relative deficit in non-anonymous sperm supply.

The law usually protects sperm donors from being responsible for children produced from their donations, and the law also usually provides that sperm donors have no rights over the children which they produce. Several countries, e.g. Sweden, Norway, the Netherlands, Britain, Switzerland, Australia and New Zealand only allow non-anonymous sperm donation. The child may, when grown up (15–18 years old), get contact information from the sperm bank about his/her biological father. In Denmark, however, a sperm donor may choose to be either anonymous or non-anonymous. Nevertheless, the initial information which the receiving woman/couple will receive is the same. In the United States, sperm banks are permitted to disclose the identity of a non-anonymous donor to any children brought to the world by that donor, once the child turns eighteen.

Where a sperm donor donates sperm through a sperm bank, the sperm bank will generally undertake a number of medical and scientific checks to ensure that the donor produces sperm of sufficient quantity and quality and that the donor is healthy and will not pass diseases through the use of his sperm. The donor's sperm must also withstand the freezing and thawing process necessary to store and quarantine the sperm. The cost to the sperm bank for such tests is not inconsiderable. This normally means that clinics may use the same donor to produce a number of pregnancies in a number of different women.

The number of children permitted to be born from a single donor varies according to law and practice. These laws are designed to protect the children produced by sperm donation from consanguinity in later life: they are not intended to protect the sperm donor himself and those donating sperm will be aware that their donations may give rise to numerous pregnancies in different jurisdictions. Such laws, where they exist, vary from state to state, and a sperm bank may also impose its own limits. The latter will be based on the reports of pregnancies which the sperm bank receives, although this relies upon the accuracy of the returns and the actual number of pregnancies may therefore be somewhat higher. Nevertheless, sperm banks frequently impose a lower limit on geographical numbers than some US states and may also limit the overall number of pregnancies which are permitted from a single donor. When calculating the numbers of children born from each donor, the number of siblings produced in any 'family' as a result of sperm donation from the same donor are almost always excluded (but see below for the provisions in various states). There is, of course, no limit to the number of offspring which may be produced from a single donor where he supplies his sperm privately.

Despite the laws limiting the number of offspring, some donors may produce substantial numbers of children, particularly where they donate through different clinics, where sperm is onsold or is exported to different jurisdictions, and where countries or states do not have a central register of donors.

Sperm agencies, in contrast to sperm banks, rarely impose or enforce limits on the numbers of children which may be produced by a particular donor partly because they are not empowered to demand a report of a pregnancy from recipients and they are rarely, if ever, able to guarantee that a woman may have a subsequent sibling by the donor who was the biological father of her first or earlier children.

Countries that have banned anonymous sperm donation have a substantial sperm shortage, because only a fraction of sperm donors want to continue their contributions if they know that the donor-conceived children may contact them one day. Banning of payment to donors has also caused shortages. This has prompted fertility tourism to other countries to get the treatment.

For instance, when Sweden banned anonymous sperm donation in 1980, the number of active sperm donors dropped from approximately 200 to 30. Sweden now has an eighteen-month-long waiting list for donor sperm. After the United Kingdom ended anonymous sperm donation in 2005, the numbers of sperm donors went up, reversing a three-year decline. However, there is still a shortage, and some doctors have suggested raising the limit of children per donor. Sperm exports from Britain are legal (subject to the EU Directive on Tissue Exports) and donors may remain anonymous in this context. Some UK clinics export sperm which may in turn be used in treatments for fertility tourists in other countries. UK clinics also import sperm from Scandinavia. Canada also has a shortage because it has been made unlawful to pay people for donating it, requiring recipients who wish to purchase it to import it from the United States. The United States, on the other hand, has had an increase in sperm donors during the late 2000s recession, with donors finding the monetary compensation more favorable.

Naturally, waiting times have gone up, and as a result more and more patients look for a donor by themselves: brothers, brothers-in-law, cousins, close friends, etc. In addition donors advertise, though this raises questions about the quality and safety of the sperm. Waiting times of almost two years also drive patients abroad to countries like Belgium, where there is still complete anonymity.

Do parents tell their children that they have been conceived with the help of a donor? With single people and lesbian couples the question doesn't arise. The greatest dilemma is whether children and sperm donor actually want to get to know each other. Suppose someone in late adolescence is told that his father is not his biological father, what will their reaction be? It's hard to imagine. Very probably few sixteen-year-olds are dying to trace their 'roots'. It would seem more obvious for them to do that when genealogical factors like birth, death, marriage or divorce come into the picture.

In my hospital donors are recruited through adverts in the regional daily newspaper. Men of 55 and over are excluded, since their generally poor sperm quality entails a higher risk of a child being born with a chromosomal abnormality. More than 80 per cent of volunteers are rejected, usually for the same reason, though occasionally a hereditary problem is grounds for rejection. Traceability and potential pressure have led to the number of families a donor may help to create being limited to five. This means that the number of times he may be approached in future is limited. The recipient of the sperm is promised that she may also have a second or subsequent child from the same donor, so that her children are true brothers and sisters. The restriction on the number of women per donor also has the advantage that the period of donorship need only be short. The men come for a period of between one and two years, every two or three weeks, in order to build up a large quantity of sperm. Of course some basic information is recorded, including height, weight, skin, eye and hair colour and certain personality features.

The sperm is released only after it has been in quarantine for six months. Meanwhile the donor has been screened again for hepatitis B and C, syphilis, chlamydia, cytomegalia and HIV. Experience has shown that the chance of a full-term pregnancy for each artificial donor insemination is approximately one in eight.

Sick sperm and original sin

'Babies Made with Sperm from Sick Donor' read the front-page headlines in the Dutch daily *Trouw* at the end of February 2002. The report that followed these striking headlines was shocking enough! Eighteen children were found to have been artificially conceived with sperm from a donor suffering from a congenital muscular disease, which had only manifested itself in the donor later in life. The chance of this being passed on was 50 per cent for each child. A nasty fright, and not just for the (foster-)parents. The report confronted the newspaper reader, just out of bed, with the alienating effects of reproductive medicine. The headline chosen only reinforced this and at any rate stayed with me, and kept buzzing through my head all that week. And certainly, the headline was 'provocative, polemical and piquant', as the editor said in justification, after extensive reader comment. 'It is a radical shock to be confronted with the downside of the "messing about" with modern reproductive techniques', wrote the editor.

'Yet that wasn't what concerned me most', wrote a very interesting magazine with a Christian perspective on faith and culture. The writer expressed his view as follows:

I have long disliked the downside of the 'messing about'. There's no need for the paper to define me with this headline. It's a little late, it seems to me. It disturbs me too. There's something hypocritical about wanting suddenly to focus in the light of this unpleasant incident on the messing-about with nature's reproductive techniques. As if when they are supposedly successful, they raise no questions. Apart from that, it is all so relative. The messing about and manipulation surrounding conception is only a special variant of the universally accepted messing and manipulation surrounding contraception. It may provoke its own moral questions, questions which are real, but to act as if natural conception in a period when contraceptives are deliberately not used is not messing about, goes too far for me. Children are not only made in laboratories, nowadays.

The headline 'Babies Made with Sperm from Sick Donor' approved by a conscientious editor concerned me because I found it an almost poetic line, reflecting as it does both modern life ('made') and the classical Calvinist teaching of man's mortal condition, or original sin ('sperm from sick donor').

And a little further:

The article casts an unusual light on something as everyday as the desire for children. It seems as if the scope and depth of the desire for children is realized precisely where this desire is not immediately fulfilled in a natural way. The fact that the desire proves to have undreamed-of highs and lows, becomes clear in the lengths people go to in order to realize their wish after all. Nether the medical route nor the adoption route are pleasant, but they are demanding, both mentally and physically. The desire is such that some people are prepared to make do with a child that is not fruit of both members of a couple.

This is in no way new. On the eve of writing I read precisely the stories of Sarah and Hannah in Genesis and Samuel. The story of Sarah in particular displays many parallels with the newspaper article. In the absence of a well-trained gynaecologist Sarah took the route of the surrogate mother. The 'fuss' casts an unusual light on such people's desire for children: honour must be saved. Without wishing to argue that the desire for children is inspired only by the desire for honour – general values (virtues) like care and love are also at issue – I would not wish to play down its importance for our age. In our children we finally transcend the finiteness and futility of our existence, perpetuate ourselves, retain our grip on the world after our death.

If in the practice of reproductive medicine you listen to what involuntarily childless couples have to say, you realize the extent to which the 'death is final' feeling can affect the ability to retain the unfulfilled desire for children. It makes everyone it affects doubly aware of human mortality. The line dies out, the name is lost. Looked at in this light, the often laborious journey through the medical circuit or the adoption mill, sometimes accompanied by moments of loss of decorum, takes on the character of a battle against the finiteness of existence. The childless couple want a share in what others regard as axiomatic.

But where awe at the mystery of procreation and sense of vulnerability are lost, or are even absent, the human soul is damaged. Parents who with the aid of assisted reproduction techniques want to 'make' a child as part of their life project, sooner or later run up against the boundaries of narcissism, certainly when a child demands a different kind of care and love than its parents had planned. Instead of blessing their child, they may come to curse it and such curses can extend a long way. If they cling to the 'project', sad self-pity is the lot they have chosen for themselves.

Vibro-ejaculation and electro-ejaculation

A spinal cord lesion is a traumatic injury to the spine. The consequences depend on the location and severity of the trauma. Fortunately it is a rare injury. It is estimated that the annual incidence of spinal cord injury (SCI), not including those who die at the scene of the accident, is approximately 40 cases per million population in the USA or approximately 11,000 new cases each year. Since there have not been any overall incidence studies of SCI in the USA since the 1970s it is not known if incidence has changed in recent years. Before the Second World War the prognosis for such people was poor, but thanks to the advance of medical science life expectancy has risen markedly and at present is only slightly a few years below the norm. The number of people in the United States who were alive in December 2003 who have SCI has been estimated to be approximately 243,000 persons, with a range of 219,000 to 279,000 persons.

Many people with a spinal cord lesion experience problems in their sex lives. Irrespective of the height of the lesion, experiencing a 'normal' orgasm is no longer possible. However a portion of spinal cord lesion patients are able to experience a form of orgasm. Often these are pleasant sensations in the transitional area between presence and absence of sensation. Possibly erratic nerve activity in the brain plays a part in this, since such activity bypasses the spinal cord.

The feeling of an orgasm is sometimes actually unpleasant, although patients turn out to experience a certain relaxation afterwards. The nerves that exit on a level with the spinal segments from the eleventh thoracic vertebra to the second lumbar vertebra (T11-L2) deal with the first part of ejaculation in men. If there is trauma above the tenth thoracic vertebra there is no more transportation of sperm, so that ejaculation is no longer possible. If there is a complete spinal lesion between T11 and L2 the results are unpredictable, depending on whether there are still impulses via this level to the epididymides, seminal ducts and seminal glands. In the case of a complete spinal cord lesion between the third lumbar vertebra and the first sacral vertebra (L3 and S1), sperm transportation and ejaculation generally remain intact.

In involuntary childlessness the poor quality of the sperm plays a role in addition to erection and ejaculation problems. The causes of this are 'accumulation' due to the lack of spontaneous ejaculation, epididymal inflammations and too high a temperature. In wheelchair patients the testicles hang more or less constantly in a warm environment.

There are various methods of treating fertility problems in cases of spinal cord lesion. If manual stimulation does not produce an ejaculation, an ordinary vibrator can be used, and if that doesn't help, a more powerful vibrator. In 80 per cent of men with a spinal cord lesion an ejaculation can be produced in this way. In individuals with a spinal cord lesion above the sixth thoracic vertebra, though, it may cause raised blood pressure and even cerebral haemorrhaging. For that reason there must be a doctor on hand, at least the first time. A similar expensive vibrator can also be used in the case of *anejaculation* with different causes, including psychological ones. Both the vibration frequency and the amplitude can be adjusted. The optimum amplitude with spinal cord lesion is 2.8 mm and a frequency of 100 Hertz. If no ejaculation can be produced with this method, the next step is electrostimulation. This involves the giving of electrical impulses via a thick probe in the rectum, causing the release of sperm cells which can subsequently be removed from the bladder. If the quality is good, the sperm cells are frozen and are used at a later date for ICSI.

This equipment was developed by vets involved in breeding programmes in zoos. In the 1970s zoos stopped capturing animals straight from the wild. An out-and-out sex and sperm tourist business developed. The sperm was obtained, with the animals under anaesthetic, by electro-ejaculation. If necessary the males went travelling. Coordinated breeding programmes monitor the reproduction of several hundred animal species of virtually all the zoos on earth. The experts look at the sex distribution, age structure and the degree of relatedness of all animals of the same type in the various parks and zoos. In this way a breeding plan is drawn up, laying down what animals may have descendants with what others.

chapter nine

Spilling One's Seed

Not so long ago, as I was walking round the Hermitage in St Petersburg, I spotted among the many paintings a wonderful etching by Rembrandt van Rijn (1606–1669) depicting a nude male model in front of a curtain. The young man is undoubtedly masturbating. Commentators speak of an 'academic posture in a classical attitude expressing balance and harmony'. I don't believe a word of it.

Male self-gratification means that the man does not inject his seed into the appropriate aperture in a female body, but wastes it. At least, for centuries this was the view of many religions. Other terms for self-gratification include masturbation, onanism and solo sex. 'Masturbation' derives from the Latin words *mas*, meaning 'manly/manliness' and *turbare*, meaning 'to move (violently)'. In reality it refers to the phenomenon that occurs in both sexes of humans and animals, namely bringing oneself through certain actions to a state of sexual arousal, whether or not followed by an orgasm, and in men the ejaculating of sperm. In Thailand they call it 'flying your kite'.

In many primates both sexes masturbate with some regularity, for example the red-capped mangabey, a soot-coloured West African monkey with a long tail and extravagant hair growth on its cheeks. And orang-utans stimulate themselves with sex toys that they make from twigs and leaves. Male red deer do it by rubbing the tips of their antlers on the grass. It takes no longer than fifteen seconds from beginning to end. Elephants of course use their trunks in masturbation.

The Romans associated masturbation with the left hand, traditionally seen as the wrong or evil hand. In general the spilling of seed has been regarded as sinful or a necessary evil. The Talmud makes no bones about it: it is forbidden to hold one's member even while urinating. There is an important linguistic distinction between masturbation and onanism. For the reader not brought up with the language of the

Rembrandt van
Rijn, *Seated Male
Nude*, 1646.

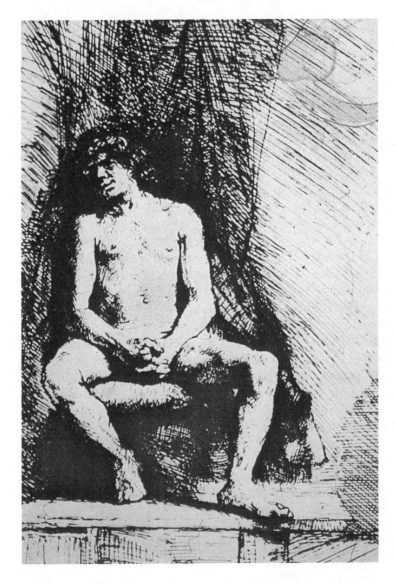

Bible, the term onanism is quite wrongly derived from Onan, a grand-son of the patriarch Jacob. In accordance with ancient Jewish custom Onan's father demanded that he marry Tamar, the widow of his dead brother and have children with her. Onan did not want to do this and so 'it came to pass, when he went in unto his brother's wife, that he spilled [his seed] upon the ground, lest that he should give seed to his brother' (Genesis 38:1–30). What Onan did is more accurately known as coitus interruptus.

Down to the nineteenth century

In the Middle Ages the Catholic church issued a long list of prohibitions in which all sins were described and assigned an appropriate penance. Masturbation scored high on this list, though the penalty imposed depended on age and marital and religious status. In the seventeenth century science adopted the conclusions of the church virtually without question, assuming that the punishment would manifest itself in disease, madness or death. One of the first alarmists was the Swiss doctor Samuel-Auguste Tissot. He regarded masturbation as a crime and an act of suicide. Haemorrhoids, constipation, epilepsy, tuberculosis, paralysis and deformed children were all consequences of this crime. One of his solutions was to sever the nerves in the penis. He wrote an academic thesis on the subject (*Traité de l'Onanisme: Dissertation sur les Maladies produites par la Masturbation*), which appeared in Latin in 1760 and in French in 1764. Unusually for a thesis, it became a best-seller, and is predictably full of amusing exaggerations.

Tissot's imitators were to make the list of symptoms and ailments caused by masturbation well-nigh endless. Various types of eye disease, headache above the eye sockets, pain at the back of the head, strange feelings above one's head, various types of neuralgia, tenderness of the skin about the lowest part of the spine, asthma, heart murmur, blisters on wounds, acne, dilated pupils, squinting, bags under the eyes, inter-mittent deafness, pale and discoloured skin, redness of the nose, rack-ing coughs, urinary incontinence, warts on the hands, a strange smell on the skin – according to the doctors these were all the result of masturbation.

In 1818 the surgeon Jalade-Lafond designed a corset for the penis. It reached from the shoulders down to the knees. Later different kinds of equipment appeared, including a metal tube which hung from a leather waistcoat, designed by the German Johann Fleck. An English in-vention perfected the German version: another metal tube was added to allow the user to urinate. The British were also responsible for naming the new diseases: *spermatorrhoia* or sexual neurasthenia. The English sexologist Havelock Ellis observed that for a highly sexed young man there was nothing for it but to enter a monastery. He devotes forty pages to this in *The Development of Morality*, which he wrote in 1897. He looks in detail at the studies published hitherto on what percentage of young men masturbated:

Brockman, also in America, among 232 theological students, of the average age of 23½ years and coming from various parts of the United States, found that 132 spontaneously admitted that masturbation was their most serious temptation and all but one of these admitted that he yielded, 69 of them to a considerable extent. This is a proportion of at least 56 per cent, the real proportion being doubtless larger, since no question had been asked as to sexual offences; 75 practiced masturbation after conversion . . .

At the end of the nineteenth century doctors believed that self-abuse, the spilling of sperm, led not only to impotence but to general debilitation. A physician wrote at the time:

The onanist is unable to perform intercourse, his member having lost the necessary resilience, the capacity to become erect.

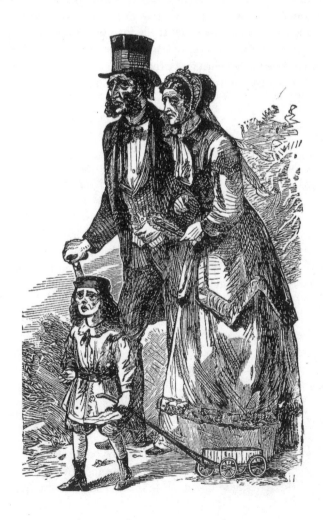

Victims of onanism.

The noble juice, his male worth, his beauty has been lost. The source from which energy, mental power, courage and pride, talent and joy sprang has dried up, it has all been recklessly spilled; perhaps a little is left, but that little is thin, watery, powerless and moreover flows from him too soon.

Underlying this kind of thinking was a theory of scarcity. This theory springs from the atavistic notion that sperm derived directly from the spinal cord. Even Leonardo da Vinci had pictured it in this way, and consequently had drawn two drainage channels in the penis, one for sperm and one for urine.

In those days, to protect boys from an erection and onanism a ring was slid over the penis before bedtime. Previously a similar device had been designed for breeding stallions. Horse breeders had always known that breeding stallions tend to self-gratification instead of waiting for a willing mare. It was a time when no deep-frozen sperm could be stored in sperm banks. Because it was thought that excessive masturbation would be to the detriment of sperm quality, a kind of net was hung over the penis, so that when the animal had an erection a bell

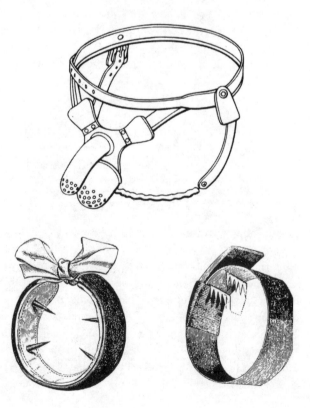

Apparatus for preventing nocturnal erections.

rang and the horse breeder could intervene urgently. The devices sold well, at eight dollars apiece, a considerable sum at that time.

William Alexander Hammond (1828–1900) a surgeon and later professor of nervous and mental diseases at New York, was also convinced that self-gratification, particularly at a young age, was the principal cause of failure to achieve an erection. In the second chapter of his book *Sexual Impotence in the Male and Female* (1887) he takes over a hundred pages to explain what he sees as the root of the problem. Organs must be 'mature' before they are put under pressure. If a child is forced to study too young, it is in serious danger of developing epilepsy or becoming an idiot. If exposed to over-strenuous physical work the child's growth will be stunted and it will remain backward and weak. For this reason Hammond is convinced that stimulation of the sex organs at an immature age leads to impotence.

As a salutary warning the professor tells the story of a young shepherd who gives himself over to onanism at a young age. Eventually the whole thing leads to gruesome complications, which are still observed in less serious form in contemporary urological practice. Throughout, the shepherd has an aversion to women. He becomes melancholy and from then on is only concerned with satisfying his desires. One day he cuts a notch with a knife right through the glans in the direction of the urethra. This operation gives him a pleasant sensation and results in an abundant ejaculation. After having repeated this gruesome mutilation a number of times, the unfortunate shepherd realizes that he has divided his penis in two from the end of the urethra to the pubic bone. Hammond continues graphically:

> When haemorrhage was particularly great, he arrested it by tying a cord around the penis. The corpora cavernosa, separated as they were, were equally capable of erection, but they diverged right and left. When the penis was divided as far as the symphysis, the knife was no longer useful . . .

New attempts and new disappointments follow:

> Among the expedients to which he resorted was one with a piece of wood shorter than the one he had previously used, and which he introduced into the part of the urethra which remained to him. He thus succeeded in exciting the very orifices of the ejaculatory ducts and in causing an emission of semen. For ten years this procedure satisfied him, until one day he was so careless in his use of his stick of wood that it escaped from his fingers and slipped into his bladder. At once he experienced

great pain, and all the efforts he made to expel the foreign body were without success. Finally after intense suffering from retention of urine and haemorrhage from the bladder, he consulted a surgeon, who was of course greatly astonished to find, instead of a single penis, two, each as large as the original. The great pain felt by the patient decided the surgeon to perform the operation of lithotomy, which having done he extracted the piece of wood – which from having been three months in the bladder was deeply encrusted with calcareous matter. After some serious drawbacks the patient recovered from the operation, but died about three months subsequently of phthisis, due to his long-continued and frequently repeated excesses.

After this anecdote you may think such things no longer happen. Well, every experienced urologist knows a patient who in solitude has tried to reach a climax by inserting an electric cord or something similar into the urethra. Usually such experiments end in a chilly operating theatre, because the cord in the urethra had started to twist.

A most unusual form of masturbation was described a few years back in a urological journal. A 40-year-old-man attended the A & E department of a hospital in Pennsylvania. His scrotum was as big as a grapefruit. The left side had been torn open and the testicle was missing. The patient said that he had been injured at work a few days earlier. When questioned further, he admitted that while his fellow workers were at lunch, he had got into the habit of holding his erect

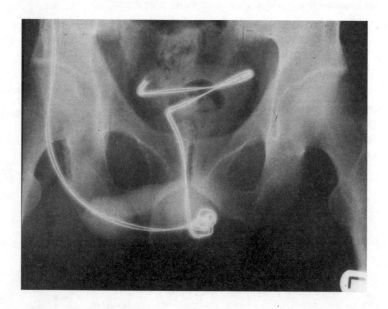

x-ray photo of an electrical cord in the urethra.

penis against a canvas drive belt of an assembly line. One day, when he was on the point of ejaculating, his scrotum became caught between the drive belt and the assembly line. The man closed the hole with eight shots from a staple gun and went gaily back to work!

In the United States there was a remarkable interest in the link between nutrition and masturbation. Both Sylvester Graham, the inventor of crackers, and John Harvey Kellogg, the inventor of corn-flakes, came up with a solution in the form of a diet. In Graham's view each ejaculation was equivalent to the loss of a considerable amount of blood, while Kellogg maintained that masturbation was even worse than sodomy. Inventors set out to find new devices to prevent mastur-bation, and between 1856 and 1932 the American authorities granted 33 patents. Meanwhile in Europe all manner of pills, syrups and medi-cines had been developed, for example, pills made of crystallized sulphuric acid and iron, syrup of lactic acid and sugar and drinks con-taining calcium chloride, magnesium chloride, sodium bicarbonate, kitchen salt, iron sulphate, sulphate of soda and carbonated water.

Ultimately neither the engineers with their apparatus, nor the doctors with their medicines, their forced sterilizations, circumcisions and committals to insane asylums, nor the Protestant or Catholic clergy could turn the tide. Incidentally it was not only Christianity that took a negative view of self-gratification. The same applied to the other two Semitic religions and, for example, Taoism. Taoism sees masturbation as pure sex – without warmth, without feeling, communication or the harmony of yin and yang. In his book *The Tao of Love and Sex* Jolan Chang writes that he is one of the few men who have masturbated no more than a dozen times in their life. 'I had the feeling that masturba-tion was too mechanical an act and that there was no poetry in it.'

The United States has produced some very enlightened scientists. Dr Alfred Kinsey saw a possible solution in large-scale research into the sexual habits of his fellow Americans, in the hope of neutralizing all kinds of sexual prejudices. He took second place when it came to written material on sex, since over the centuries the Vatican remained unsurpassed. Kinsey produced more than eight thousand case histories, in which 88 per cent of those questioned between the ages of sixteen and twenty turned out to indulge in self-gratification. Less than half a century later Shere Hite produced her *Hite Report on Male Sexuality*. She noted that many men feel guilty during masturbation, but at the same time derive great pleasure from it.

Modern views

By the way, the above stories are certainly not meant to imply that masturbation is an unhealthy form of sex. On the contrary, modern sexologists see it as a form of sperm quality control: in that way it can never become old and over-ripe. Truman Capote said the interesting thing about masturbation was that he didn't have to get dolled up for it, and even fifty years ago a popular American professor was telling his students that masturbation had many advantages: 'It saves time and money, it avoids quite a few unhappy relationships and obligations, it makes no one unhappy and there is no risk of infectious diseases.' The Hollywood director Woody Allen hit the nail on the head with his quip: 'Don't knock masturbation – it's sex with someone I love.' However, all in all it's not very sensible, for example, to masturbate five times in quick succession: the seminal glands will empty and eventually all that will come out is a little fluid, or in the worst case blood.

Internet sites like www.nowscape.com list literally hundreds of slang terms for (male) masturbation in addition to the 'standard' terms 'wank' (UK) and 'jerk off' (US). Some the more inventive euphemisms include:

> assault on a friendly weapon, beating your meat, being your own best friend, charm the cobra, couch hockey for one, cranking the shank, Custer's last stand, disseminating, flogging your dong, getting in touch with your manhood, hand job, holding all the cards, manual override, one-handed clapping, peel the carrot, playing with Dick, play the stand-up organ, pocket pool, popping the porpoise, pull off, pumping for pleasure, punishing Percy, ride the great white knuckler, rope the pony, rounding up the tadpoles, self love, shaking hands with the governor, shooting Sherman, slammin' the salami, slap-boxing the one-eyed champ, spanking your monkey, squeeze the lemon, walking the dog, whacking off, whipping the pony, winding the jack-in-a-box, etc, etc.

The activity features frequently in song lyrics, for example in Jethro Tull's teasingly ambiguous 'Roll Yer Own':

> Roll yer own, roll it when there's something missing
> and those wild cats howl, running in the moonshine.
> Roll yer own if you can't buy readymade; you won't be satisfied
> when you feel the sudden need to unwind.
> Roll yer own: you got to hit that spot.
> Roll yer own when your hands are hot.

In novels, though one can find plenty about sexual dissipation, masturbation does not usually figure prominently. In English-language fiction the great exception is Philip Roth's classic *Portnoy's Complaint* (1969), whose protagonist's sexual obsessions, and specifically his compulsive masturbation, reflect his revolt against his parents, his Jewishness and social injustice.

In his *Confessions* Jean-Jacques Rousseau chronicles his lonely battle with masturbation:

> I learned this dangerous supplement which deceives nature and leads young men of my disposition to many excesses at the expense of their health, their vigour and sometimes even of their lives. This vice, which shame and timidity find so convenient, is, moreover, particularly attractive to active imaginations: it allows them to dispose at will, say, of the entire female sex, and to make a tempting beauty serve their pleasures without needing to obtain her consent.

The Russian writer Nikolai Vasilyevich Gogol (1809–1852), perhaps best known for his *Diary of a Madman*, was an extravagant masturbator, which was undoubtedly connected with his melancholy disposition, and the same was true of the Danish philosopher Sören Kierkegaard. Masturbation was actually the preferred form of love-making of the English poet Philip Larkin ('Love again: wanking at ten past three'). He had diffident relationships with women, never wanted to marry, disliked children and defined sex as 'one of those social activities that worlds removed from me, like playing baccarat or clog-dancing'. For most of his rather solitary life he was librarian of the University of 'dull Hull', which suited him down to the ground.

It has even been said of Goethe that when young he frequently 'took matters into his own hands', probably prompted by a passage in *Truth and Fiction*, in which he describes his student life in Leipzig. He loses his sweetheart there because, so he believes, he has neglected her. He relates how he took his frustration out on his own body:

> I had lost her really; and the frenzy with which I revenged my fault upon myself, by assaulting in various frantic ways my physical nature, in order to inflict some hurt on my moral nature, contributed very much to the bodily maladies under which I lost some of the best years of my life: indeed, I should perchance have been completely ruined by this loss, had not my poetic talent here shown itself particularly helpful with its healing power.

Does everyone do it?

In the media it is claimed that everyone does it, but that's not true. Scientific research by G. Van Zessen and T. Sandfort published in 1991 showed that 18 per cent of men and 45 per cent of women never masturbate.

Nowadays most sex manuals suggest that masturbation is a good way of discovering your own body, and helps an adolescent to be better prepared when he or she starts having sex with a partner. This implies that masturbation is fine, but unnecessary once one has a relationship.

Based on changes in sexual attitudes in the last few decades it is assumed that in general masturbation no longer poses a problem. However, large-scale surveys among young people of upbringing, sexuality and early childhood experiences reveal that just under half of young people under sixteen have had concerns about it, occasionally or more often. Analysis of interview clips shows that the concerns can be grouped in four categories: guilt feelings, fear of disease, and doubts and uncertainty due to ignorance. These categories can easily be traced back to the traditional myths about masturbation. All this takes place against a background awareness that, in short, solo sex is becoming more and more popular. Who could have imagined thirty years ago that the sexual revolution would implode into mass masturbation at one's own computer? Only forty years ago many boys were ticked off when their mothers had trouble getting their sheets clean. How many of those parents, themselves brought up as children of the sexual revolution, prepare their own sons or daughters for what awaits them in puberty with a nice friendly chat? That might prevent a few years of guilt feelings. Why not simply say that masturbation is a 'normal' activity?

In *A Conspiracy of Dunces* the American writer John Kennedy Toole (1937–1969) describes how pleasant and satisfying it can be. The novel is set in New Orleans and tells the story of Ignatius J. Reilly, an unforgettable, Quixotic protagonist: overweight, burping, terrorizing those around him intellectually. His insufferably arrogant character, together with the unimaginable aura of bodily odours than envelops him, has not brought him much success in job interviews. But when he does land a job at Levy Pants, he organizes a wildcat strike and is fired; he ends up as a hotdog seller. John Kennedy Toole committed suicide at the age of 32, and *A Conspiracy of Dunces* appeared posthumously in 1980, thanks to the efforts of the author's mother. In the following passage Ignatius reflects on the place of masturbation in his life:

Ignatius touched the small erection that was pointing down-ward into the sheet, held it, and lay still trying to decide what to do. In this position, with the red flannel nightshirt around his chest and his massive stomach sagging into the mattress, he thought somewhat sadly that after eighteen years with his hobby it had become merely a mechanical physical act stripped of the flights of fancy and invention that he had once been able to bring to it. At one time he had almost developed it into an art form, practicing the hobby with the skill and fervor of an artist and philosopher, a scholar and a gentleman.

A survey of 2003 showed that for both men and women in the area of sexual taboos, self-gratification stands incontestably at number one. Erection problems and sexually transmitted diseases were at numbers two and three respectively. Women tend to talk more openly but in the case of masturbation they find it more difficult than men (47% as opposed to 32%). Masturbation is certainly not a standard topic of conversation. Is it perhaps that there is so little of interest to be said about it? One may wonder if it comes under the heading of sex at all. For a while it was fashionable in America to tell young people in sex manuals that masturbation is a safer option than sex. This is a sop to sweeten a recommendation of abstinence, and of course it doesn't work. One activity has simply nothing to do with the other. Whatever one may understand by sex, it is at least something social, while masturbation goes in the direction of private grooming activities like picking scabs or squeezing spots.

Taboos are things one doesn't talk about with others in one's immediate environment, either because one is ashamed or because it isn't done to talk about them. The respondents in the above-mentioned survey were also asked what taboo in modern society should no longer be a taboo. And the result in respect of masturbation? Only 8 per cent of women and 16 per cent of men felt the taboo should go. Conclusion: the taboo on masturbation will therefore remain. Is that so terrible? I don't think so. When all's said and done, a little sperm does get spilt. And don't let's forget the trees felled for the millions of paper tissues!

'Can masturbation harm you? No. Does it do you good? Just for a second. But apart from that it's a rather silly occupation,' as a colum-nist once put it. 'Silly – like wolfing down a cake or a snack – and call-ing it supper.' Who's to argue with her?

chapter ten

Women

As a remedy against the temptations of the flesh the Buddhists devised a meditation in which they imagined woman's body as a bag of filth. Medieval ascetics viewed woman as 'a temple built above a sewer', and St Augustine said: 'Woman is the gate of hell.' If one takes these words literally many men have entered hell down the ages, at any rate too many for them all to be damned. Perhaps it is precisely those who failed to enter the gate who wind up there. Perhaps the abstainers have most to hide, who is to say?

Abnormalities at the gate

Certain physical abnormalities in the woman – abnormalities at the gate – can cause impotence. J. Smit, in his *Manual for Men and Women Suffering from Impotence, Infertility and Other Mechanical Sexual Disorders* (1810), formulates the problem as follows:

> Aristotle is right: fat ladies have too little charm, are too cold-blooded, their ovaries, encased in excessive fat, complicate the release of an ovum, the plastic lymph is too sticky and in addition the fat belly with its mass of bulging lard-like foothills prevents the male member from penetrating deeply enough. Lean food, exercise, gardening, short periods of sleep, and mental activity is the best advice. Mustard, although it is the most powerful agent for melting fat away, has too great a weakening effect on the digestive system, breaks down calcium in the blood to too great an extent, and becomes detrimental to health.
>
> Meanwhile examples have frequently been seen of portly ladies giving birth to several children; however, they find child-

birth very hard. For the rest, a *cul de Paris*, or a well-stuffed cushioned pillow, can provide a great deal of relief.

Too narrow a vagina, natural or acquired, can also cause problems. When a gynaecologist operates on a prolapse, he or she will make sure that the vagina remains at least two fingers wide, the approximate thickness of the average penis. Smit wrote of the naturally narrow vagina:

> Too narrow a sheath, as is sometimes found in very delicate, thin women, makes intercourse painful, unpleasant and fruit-less. In one case, where after several attempts over nine months the well-endowed man was able to penetrate only as far as the glans, the couple were obliged by pain on both sides to cease all further attempts. Dr Thilenius ordered an injection of almond oil morning and evening and left an easily extractable, four-inch-long piece of sponge, which had been coated with oil, in the vagina.
>
> Men who are equipped with an exceptionally strong glans, may be congenial to women of experience, but until deflora-tion, for the pleasure of young innocent girls, they are very unsuited. If the young husband encounters such a distressing situation, it is permissible for him to prepare the way with his finger.

With his surfeit of male sex hormone and high stress levels the man lives on average a few years less than the woman. Many men are dependent on a woman not only for their birth, but also for geriatric care. An unknown Englishman once wrote: 'Without this good friend [the woman] the dawn and evening of life would be helpless, and its mid-day without pleasure.'

Women receive the fertilizing sperm, help the embryo develop and bear our children. However you put it, reproduction is closely linked to love, loving, sexuality. In all kinds of ways women are *the* experts.

Not so long ago some women in the Bandjoema tribe had an important role to play in this respect. Before a young man was granted the right to marry, he had to take a sexual exam. The young man had to prove that in marriage he would be able to do his reproductive duty. The female examiner, called a *sentondang*, had to give a report to the father. Such reports were usually formulated as follows: 'Father, your son is a complete man.' If she did not consider the test successful and wanted a 'resit', she said: 'Father, I can't say much yet.' What wisdom in such a culture! Things are very different with some Western women.

My former partner once told me very vividly how her grandmother prized the sexual performance of her grandfather, who was then nearly eighty. Granny said: 'He still wants it every week, but there's not much left, you know. He almost has to shove it in with a fork.'

A former GP told me about a very respectable widower who late in life met a strapping Flemish woman. He married her, but unfortunately he proved to be impotent. Time after time she made fun of him and belittled him to his face. On one occasion she said: 'Shall I do a handstand, so you can hang it in there.' The GP referred the man to a famous sexologist, with a letter of referral in which he wrote that the wife was 'stiffening his lack of resolve'. Of course there are also men who talk deprecatingly about their wife's genitals. Generations of feminism and political correctness have not yet ousted 'cunt' as a term of abuse (for both sexes) in English.

The art of seduction

In our culture many men tend to 'instrumentalize' sexuality: they concentrate on certain parts of the body rather than the whole woman. Women generally focus more on the man as a 'person', and the vast majority find it hard to give themselves unless they have been touched emotionally. One cannot say it often enough: in contrast to what men may think, most women are basically not that interested in the penis, not even in that of their sexual partner. No more than a third find the dimensions of the penis important and then, whatever men may think, what matters is the girth, not the length. The crucial thing is that the glans should be clean. Some women, whether lesbian or not, have long since replaced the penis with a pipette full of sperm. 'Penis-centred' men – known in sexological jargon as 'pistils' – do not interest them at all. Strangely enough, in the plant world pistils are female and stamens male!

Modern men are rather poor at seduction, at the ritual of courtship that precedes lovemaking. Going straight up to a woman and telling her you think she's sexy, a turn-on, fit, etc., isn't seduction. Nor is deluging her with love letters, phone calls, bunches of flowers or invitations to candlelit dinners. Nor are long walks on the beach, although it is beginning to look like it. In the 1990s a gay newspaper summed up the ideal (for gays?):

> It is letting desire develop, like a slowly germinating plant, the seed of which was planted without anyone noticing. Then you cultivate that desire, water the plant, but ensure that there is still an edge of thirst. You let it grow, fertilize it, prune it and

whisper sweet words to the emerging blossom, and all without the plant knowing. Then, when the day has arrived, the bud bursts open and the flower turns towards the light. And lo and behold: the plant comes towards you, it gyrates with pleasure on your windowsill and offers you everything that you could never have obtained by asking. That is real seduction.

The psychologist Erick Janssen asked both male and female test subjects to put a number of 'separate' components of a lovemaking session in what they considered to be the normal order: stroking of the breasts, removing underpants/panties, kissing, undoing bra, intercourse, fellatio, etc. The replies of men and women, as expected, corresponded almost exactly. Next the subjects were asked to give the separate components a rating, indicating the degree of arousal per component. It was found that in men the degree of arousal ran in parallel with the 'normal' order (on which men and women were agreed). With the female test subjects, however, this was not the case: with components where in accordance with the 'normal' sequence they were expected to do something with the penis (take your pick), the arousal level plunged! It would appear that most women are really not that interested.

So is the penile erection redundant? No! Though one might almost be inclined to think so, especially when reading women's magazines, according to which women have a distinct preference for men who are both empathetic and good listeners. They adore household chores and the children, while remaining sexually faithful and in bed are devoted to their wives. They have a natural aversion to porn and aggression, feel no need for power and attach no importance to winning or being proved right. In short: a pretty weird collection of qualities for the average man. The articles confirm the stereotypical image that women do not go for strong, potent men. Intercourse, they would have us believe, scores very low on the female list of priorities. The journalist Sarah Verroen believes that is all nonsense. She conducted her own TV survey on the ideal lover. Thirty women from the fields of art, science, journalism and prostitution were approached about taking part in this – it must be said, totally unrepresentative – mini-survey.

The results were striking. In answer to the question of what women found most satisfying sexually, 29 of the 30 women put a cross against 'a good, hard fuck', and one chose 'extended lovemaking with lots of attention to my needs', while no one found 'vanilla sex' appealing. 24 of the 30 wanted 'bold, knows what he wants and what you want', 'dominant and a bit of a brute' had five crosses against it, while 'tender and completely focused on your desires' was chosen by only one woman. Verroen decries the wishy-washy taste of vanilla sex and makes it clear that at least some women are in favour of making love with men with a firm erection, of the phallus with its male attributes of effectiveness, power and penetration. In her view eroticism exists by the grace of generosity: it is the smouldering flame that unexpectedly catches fire.

The new impotence

In the early 1970s there was talk of the 'new' impotence. Partly because of advances in medical science in the preceding two decades the 1970s were to be the age in which the women's movement would demand equal sexual rights. Women began making demands on intercourse. It wasn't a matter of quantity as it had been for the Queen of Aragon (who demanded sex six times a day), but of quality. The annoying thing was that many men proved unable to cope and replied with impotence. The world gradually became feminized, and women started laying down the rules. Some men no longer knew what it meant to be a man, and became totally confused. Some of feminist demands were indeed baffling. One moment the man had to overpower the woman, but the next caress her tenderly. But, and here comes the crunch, the man had to intuit for himself when to adopt which strategy:

> For that moment when they enter Ela, men feel in control, for it is their erection which excites her. That glory evaporates as they get busy deciding what tempo to follow, which parts of her body are most sensitive, how to use their muscles, weight, skin and memory to satisfy her, how long it takes her to come, how to time their orgasm to coincide with hers. They blank out their pleasure to concentrate on hers. They delay their sensations and carefully plan to start with a bit of finger and tongue.

This is how Greek-born feminist Eurydice Kamvisseli puts it in her novel *F/32* (1990).

Like today's liberated women, medieval witches, as previously mentioned, were accused of causing impotence. They did it with a ligature. That is, the art of putting a knot in the lace of a man's breeches which led the man to become impotent through a kind of transferable magic. Preferably it should be done at the time the marriage was celebrated. This involved the witch pronouncing a magic formula, after which the lace was hidden. At the same time the witch threw two coins over her shoulder, as a symbol of the disabled testes. The impotence continued until the unfortunate victim found the lace, failing which the impotence was permanent.

In the seventeenth century this ritual provoked such violent terror in certain areas of France that many couples had their marriage solemnized at night or in a neighbouring village, in order to avoid the knotting of the lace. The seventeenth-century Dutch poet and moralist Jacob Cats mentions in his *Touchstone for the Wedding Ring* how a certain Martin Guerre 'was incapable for a full eight or nine years of paying his wife the due attentions; and that because of certain evil arts that in France are called the knotted lace'. Witches could also bring about impotence with the aid of magic potions, and could reverse the process in the same way, making them excellent sex therapists.

Undoubtedly the same applies to today's liberated women: men badly need these modern witches! It is no longer the case that men are keener on sex than their female partners, or that women stare at the ceiling and make mental shopping lists during sex. Women want an orgasm, preferably two or three in succession, the way the women's magazines promise them so temptingly. 'And this is precisely when men are more and more often turning off in bed, and would sooner bury their head in a book than in her bosom,' as a feminist once wrote.

In feminist confessional literature men generally take quite a beating. The novelist Erica Jong, in her bestselling *Fear of Flying*, exorcizes her penis envy and emphasizes the fantastic qualities of the female genitalia in contrast. She turns a 'spineless guy' into a 'spineless prick', a cruel description she uses repeatedly. Erica maintains that she has been a feminist all her life, but her biggest problem is to reconcile her feminism with her insatiable hunger for male bodies, which proves far from easy. In addition it becomes increasingly clear that men are basically terrified of women, some secretly, others openly. What could be more poignant than an emancipated woman eye to eye with a limp prick. In her eyes the major issues of history pale beside the two essential facts: the eternal feminine and the eternal limp prick. A typical fragment:

> The ultimate sexist put-down: the prick that lies down on the job. The ultimate weapon in the war between the sexes: the limp prick. The banner of the enemy's encampment. The symbol of the apocalypse: the atomic warhead prick which self-destructs. *That* was the basic inequality which could never be righted: not that the male had a wonderful added attraction called a penis, but that the female had a wonderful all-weather cunt. Neither storm nor sleet nor dark of night could faze it. It was always there, always ready. Quite terrifying, when you think about it. No wonder that men hated women. No wonder they invented the myth of female inadequacy.

Erica Jong takes a very sharp and humourless view of male impotence. Not very cheering for a man – but then that probably was her intention.

As has been said, taking the initiative sexually is no longer the prerogative of the man. These days women make demands which their partner simply has to meet. Some direct their bedfellows as if they were football coaches: stroke me a bit more to the left, a bit harder, a bit softer, etc. In the past the man called the tune in bed, and the woman more or less complied, but today's woman is not content for her partner to ejaculate after a few minutes and then roll over on his side. In the view of some experts women's demands lead to ambivalence and uncertainty about male identity. Be that as it may, the fact remains that according to influential sexologists some men even today don't like sex with the woman on top! Man's sexual emancipation has only just begun!

If he's not in the mood

According to recent American research 40 per cent of men don't feel much like sex and regard lovemaking with their partner as a duty, more work than play. It is no accident that the first self-help manual on this nettlish topic recently appeared in the United States. 'Making sure you're properly equipped' plays an important part in it, but that is easier said than done. There is also a career to be worked at, a mortgage to repay. Eating out and sports club membership are expensive, and you have to pay for all that.

It may also be that the man has gone off the idea because his wife has got a promotion and not only earns more but also works longer hours so that he has to 'hold the fort' at home. Or that the man loses his urge because they have to do it every Saturday night, when he's tired. Only stands to reason, doesn't it, after a hard week at work, people over on Saturday evening, when he has to get up early Sunday morning to go jogging with the guy next door?

The enlightened feminist Yvonne Kroonenberg (1951–) explains in her book *Alles went behalve een vent* (You Can Get Used to Anything Except a Man, 1990) why postmodern man may sometimes not be in the mood. In her view it is open to question whether men are that horny or whether they just say they are. She knows plenty of women who complain of the reverse. She tells Anke's story. Anke is married to Henk, a heavily built, pleasant guy, who prefers playing about with his computer to playing about with his wife. They had been to doctors, so-called sexologists, who suspected obscure inhibitions in his sexual feelings. But Henk shrugged his shoulders and said:

An orgasm is nice, but it's such a business getting there. I don't enjoy just banging away at Anke, so to create a party atmosphere, I need to stroke her and make sure she comes. Only then do I want to fuck and I don't like the idea of going straight off to sleep afterwards, so we have a little afterplay. It's all great fun, but not something for every day.

Another man tells the author that he has a big problem with 'objectivity'. When he's with a woman, he observes himself. He sees his white buttocks going up and down and is always mortified. That's why he'd rather stop altogether . . .

The fact remains, though, that women can also be partly responsible for the man's erection problems. A slovenly appearance, bad breath and excessive hair growth are all factors that can lead to male impotence. The nineteenth-century doctor Smit, mentioned above, formulated the problem as follows:

> A scolding, bad-tempered woman can make a man so cool that he loses the desire to fulfil his marital duties, and he gradually becomes incapable of intercourse with her. Revulsion at messiness, dislike of particular things, can extinguish the effect for particular people, sometimes gradually, sometimes suddenly. Women and girls who do not keep their bodies clean, whose private parts exude a strong, unpleasant odour, or whose breath is bad, who neglect to wash their feet, particularly when they sweat heavily, etc. often become the objects of aversion and disgust. Someone who was keen to embrace a woman of pleasure, saw a louse running over her body, and immediately became impotent. Another heard a girl making water, and was forced to leave without finishing his business. With a third a feeling of embarrassment produced the same effect. He was in the full vigour of his youth, and fully prepared to enjoy a common whore. But the latter conceived the idea of checking her lovers' health in advance, and wanted to see his manhood. The young man, as yet unfamiliar with such behaviour, found it so strange that his vigour turned instantly to impotence.

If a man develops erection problems, for instance because he has lost his job or has learned that he is infertile, the key to the solution of the problem is the way his partner reacts. The modern view is that women are just as responsible for the success of intercourse as men. This contrasts with the beginning of the twentieth century, when sexologist Premsela wrote the following:

Sexually, every woman achieves what her husband makes of her. He – and he alone is her teacher in this. That education requires time and knowledge, and in the first instance time. I read somewhere that the honeymoon of the copper wedding in a good marriage is better than that of an ordinary wedding.

In this respect husband and wife are unequal partners and it is principally the man – the leader in the sexual relationship – who must take account of this fact. He must not jump the gun and must realize that he can only achieve results gradually.

Premsela is quite persuasive, but the reverse is equally true: sexually every man achieves what his wife is able to make of him. Several centuries ago the French surgeon Nicolas Venette (1633–1698) summarized the situation in a single sentence: 'If a woman's hand does not succeed in making the penis stiff, no other treatment will be successful . . .'.

The twenty-first century

Unfortunately as far as 'seduction' is concerned the twenty-first century has begun as a time of confusion and there is no immediate sign of improvement. Now male reluctance to show emotions has been overcome, the 'new' post-feminist woman turns out to have had enough of cotton wool. Men must again, as they have traditionally done, fight back their tears. There are no more certainties. There was always one aspect that supported men through difficult times. As a man you could always rely on it, and that put you beyond women's reach: sex and love were never confused. Having sex and being in love at the same time was a kind of bonus. In most cases what young men experienced was an unbridled hunger for sex. Good sex, bad sex, emotionless one-night sex, it didn't matter. The sole performance criterion was a single feeling: lust.

There has been an obvious sea change. Nowadays the young generation of women have sex for sex's sake. Today's young women are self-confident, assertive, promiscuous and brazen. After the sexual revolution, heralded by the pill, the waves of feminism and the achievement of economic independence, for the time being woman, with her much greater social intelligence, still has the initiative. The man as hunter – those were the days. Women worldwide watched the TV hit *Sex and the City* in their thousands. Not only were viewers being presented with four highly educated single women, but the really revolutionary thing was the unbridled pursuit of a great deal of high-quality sex by PR executive Samantha Jones. Keep your wedding plans! Samantha prefers pleasure to love and is proud of it! True, this was a frequent component of many TV series and films in previous decades, but then it was always a male prerogative. The man's role has shifted: from active to passive. Will it all come right in the end? I have my doubts!

Jean de La Fontaine (1621–1695), a member of the Académie Française and best known for his animal fables, also wrote much erotic poetry, including the following 'Epigram':

> Let's Love, let's Fuck, these are pleasures
> That one must never separate;
> Enjoyment and lust are rare treasures
> For the soul to cultivate.
> A Prick, a Cunt, and two fond hearts
> Create sweet songs in many parts,
> Which the holy wrongly blame.
> Amaryllis, ponder this:
> Love without sex is a paltry flame,
> Sex without love is empty bliss.

chapter eleven

Eroticism

Erection, orgasm and reproduction form part of a long cycle, in which people partially fade into the background as they pass on their life to their descendants. In the last analysis we live not only for ourselves, but partly also for previous and succeeding generations. Seen in this light, intercourse, having an orgasm and fathering descendants is experiencing a thousand centuries in an instant. The most innovative presentation of the significance of all this was that of Georges Bataille (1897–1962), one of the founder-members of the Surrealist movement. In Bataille's view mankind's whole journey, from a monocellular micro-organism to *Homo sapiens erectus*, is actually an erection in itself. Yet he sees that erection as incomplete, since man's eyes are parallel to the earth and are still not able to withstand the sight of their ultimate goal, the dazzling sun.

Bataille was obsessed by atheism, eroticism and mysticism. He engaged in psychoanalysis, economics, philosophy and sociology. He wrote poetry, novels, studies on ethnology, the visual arts and literature. God, sex and death remained his principal themes. In *Visions of Excess* Bataille explains that mankind's mission will have been fulfilled when the pineal gland in the front of our forebrain opens and the content of the human body pours out in an ejaculation towards the sun. In his view this will be the logical conclusion of human evolution. The link that Bataille makes between the sun and sexuality is not totally ridiculous. When in spring the days grow longer and blossoms appear all over, many hearts beat faster. More sunshine has a particular effect on the brain: the production of melatonin, a hormone that inhibits sexuality, is reduced.

Computer sex

A professor of neuroanatomy at Groningen University is convinced that all sexual behaviour can be explained with the aid of brain scans and computer models. 'As long as you programme computers properly, of course you can teach them to fuck,' were his actual words. His statement testifies to an ancient and outdated view of mankind, the mechanistic vision of the Enlightenment. The professor's ideas lead to a worldview in which man is seen as nothing more than tissue, cells, molecules, atoms, elementary particles, whose behaviour is laid down in natural laws. Everything that makes us human – cultures, values and standards – falls outside the hard natural sciences. For a true understanding of human sexuality, the humanities are much more important, for example literary studies. In 1928 Bataille published the novella *History of the Eye* under a pseudonym. It is a gruesome book, which does not allow the reader to assume a voyeuristic role, but makes him, so to speak, complicit in a series of crimes. The book shows clearly that by breaking bounds sexuality turns into violence and from violence into death. Bataille calls orgasm *le petit mort*. In the little death there is a longing for the great death, the totally other, that might cancel out man's dreadful existence. The central paradox is that man is only truly human in a desire that drives him to inhumanity.

Bataille spent a long time in psychoanalysis, which made him aware of the unconscious mechanisms that influence human thought processes. In his work Freud showed how associations often operated through the sound of words, and in the novella Bataille associates *oeil* (eye) with *oeuf* (egg). The identical initial sound 'oe' may have been the reason why he looked for similarities in meaning: eyes and eggs are round and white. In another associative leap he links eye and testicle. In the sentence where he makes the link he manages to make the two resemble each other in sound too. He speaks of 'testi*cules*' and 'globe o*cul*aire'. The shared word *cul* means cunt or arse in French. Curiously, he goes on to make this a keyword, using it as a synonym for 'cunt'. In so doing he links the anal and the genital, and a little further on eye, egg and urine. There follows a disturbing confusion of all bodily orifices and all types of fluids: eye – egg – testicle – breast – arse, which secrete tears – sperm – milk – shit – and urine. They can also be destroyed in all kinds of ways: dug out – broken – removed by castration – drunk – severed and deflowered. Because the egg equals the testicle, the female protagonist can satisfy her desire to castrate by crushing an egg between her legs, and because the testicle equals the egg, she can eat the former raw instead of the latter, and because the eye equals the testicle she can stick the eye up her arse, etc. The characters produce a series of metaphors. For example, the woman rolls an egg across her vulva, later she sticks a bull's testicle in her vagina and finally also a priest's eye. All these acts are obscene parodies of 'normal' intercourse. Georges Bataille, like Sigmund Freud before him, demonstrates clearly that man is potentially a polymorphously perverse creature.

Sexologists

The first sexologists were still heavily influenced by Victorian thinking. Havelock Ellis, an English doctor, was the first Victorian with a modern view of sexuality. He believed that a person's attitude to sexuality was individually and culturally determined. This was something totally new, since in the preceding centuries, it had been assumed that sex was the same for everyone.

The contribution of Sigmund Freud will be familiar to many readers. He gave a name to the unconscious and classified the sexual components of our personality. Freud was one of the first doctors to listen to his patients, and was the first to point out how important it is for the patient to gain an insight into his or her own problems. Theodoor Hendrik van de Velde (1873–1937), a Dutch gynaecologist, made an important contribution to sexology. His international best-seller *The Perfect Marriage* (1926) is one of the most famous modern sex manuals, selling over a million copies. Van de Velde stressed the importance of sexual relations and an attitude of giving and taking. Unfortunately he limited his readers' sexual experience by advocating that they should strive where possible for simultaneous orgasm – an over-romantic presentation of the facts. In that respect manuals sometimes do more harm than good. For a long time Van de Velde remained a classic example of a prophet without honour in his own country, and it is not difficult to guess why. He wrote frankly about desire and sex, which, in those days at least, was not done. What's more he ran off with one of his patients, a married woman eight years his junior – another no-no.

In America it was Robert Latou Dickinson who did ground-breaking work, also with women. For example, he examined the vagina with the aid of a glass tube in the shape of a penis, through which a lamp could be shone. This allowed him to observe the interior of the vagina directly, and this aid was refined by later researchers.

Alfred Kinsey, who had trained as a zoologist, did mainly large-scale quantitative research into human sexuality. Though many 'case histories' had been written, especially by Freudians, no one had ever used large samples. Certain sexual practices today regarded as perfectly normal were considered 'deviant' by the Freudians. Kinsey demon-

strated that much 'abnormal' sexual behaviour, for example homosexuality, is in fact quite normal.

William Masters (1915–2001) and Virginia Johnson (1925–) were
the founders of modern sexology, a typical interdisciplinary science.
They had the courage to observe and measure sexual responses in the
same way that physiologists had studied respiration or digestion.
Masters determined at the outset of his scientific work that he would
collaborate with a woman since he as a man would never be able to
understand how a woman experiences sexuality. This was a brilliant
idea. In the treatment of men with erection problems, the reverse may
be true: only men can fully understand what a man feels in such a case.
Masters and Johnson achieved overnight fame when they published
their first book, *Human Sexual Inadequacy* (1966). 'Older couples can
enjoy a healthy, normal sex life, at least well into their eighties,' wrote
Time, and there was a general chorus of approval from the media.

Masters and Johnson's idea was that a couple where the man had
erection problems, should spend more time together, say on two
evenings a week. On one evening it was the man's responsibility to
create the right mood, and on the other the woman's, preferably with
background music and tasty nibbles and dips. And then the couple,
naked on the sofa, were supposed to stroke each other a little, though
the man had to stay above the belt! The intention was to take sexuality out of the sphere of emotional rejection, the urge to perform and the
fear of failure. In a number of cases the therapy proved effective. Probably it was connected with what we used to call 'tag-free' in games of
hide and seek: if you stood on a certain spot, you couldn't be tagged.
Some women felt 'tag-free' in this therapy since the rules of the exercise
did not allow them to be touched below the belt. A bit of back rubbing,
that was all – very primitive, in fact, but sometimes it worked.

If that didn't help, one could do a course of therapy at the Masters
and Johnson clinic. For the treatment of impotent bachelors they had
secured the assistance of female volunteers, who were carefully chosen.
The therapy had three main aims: the man must rid himself of his fear
of failure, and of the habit of playing the observer and the woman must
regain confidence in her man. These aims were to be achieved by means
of emotional concentration exercises. Just as at home, the couples were
not initially allowed to have intercourse, only stroking and caressing,
so they had no need to fear failure. The man usually achieved an erection after one or two of these sessions. At this stage the couple were still
not allowed to have intercourse, but had to continue the pleasurable
stroking until erections occurred regularly. Then the couples had to
practise making the erection disappear and come back again. The
idea was that the man should overcome his fear that if the erection

disappeared during intercourse, it would not return at all. When the experts felt that the moment had come to tell the man to attempt to penetrate the vagina, the woman was instructed to kneel over her partner. She had to insert the penis into the vagina and make sure that at that stage she made no demands. If the erection disappeared she was to make the penis erect again with her hand. This treatment by Masters and Johnson proved successful with over 60 per cent of men.

Their treatment methods came in for their fair share of criticism. One of the objections was that the human aspects of sexual intercourse were neglected. In the view of the critics Masters and Johnson saw coitus too much as a kind of mechanical process of stimulation and responses. They were accused of paying insufficient attention to the spiritual element in human sexual experience. Yet for all the criticism these two sexologists retain their reputation as pioneers in their field.

As regards scientific research into erection problems, Erick Janssen made a significant contribution in 1995, distinguishing between the *reflex* erection and the arbitrary *psychogenic* erection. The first type operates through the spinal column and results from touching or stimulation of the penis. The psychogenic erection originates in the brain and in response to visual impulses, erotic fantasies, etc. Scarcely any research had been done on how the two sorts of erection combine and interact. Janssen provided a research structure with which the interplay could be studied. Men with ED were exposed to physical and visual erotic stimuli, separately or in combination. For physical stimulation he used a ring-shaped vibrator that could be slid over the penis. The visual stimuli consisted of erotic film clips. It was found that with test subjects whose ED had been diagnosed in the old way as probably psychological in nature, the purely physical stimulus of the vibrator scarcely resulted in an erection. If the men simultaneously watched an erotic film, an erection was achieved much more easily – as if concerns about one's own sexual functioning affected mainly the reflex erection. When the erotic film was added, these concerns could obviously be suppressed and the physical experience – the vibration of the penis – could be placed more in a sexual context.

The fact that negative experiences or sexual worries can impede the achieving of an erection was shown by the following. If the impotent men were asked while watching the erotic film to do mental arithmetic or to watch a Tom and Jerry cartoon, the erection achieved turned out to be stronger. Mental arithmetic and cartoon mice can obviously reduce erection problems!

In addition Janssen believes that, in contrast to what is claimed, fear of failure is *not* a cause of impotence. Research shows that this claim by no means always holds good. For example, a number of test subjects were asked to achieve an erection within two minutes, or they would be given an electric shock. 'The shocks were never given,' said Janssen, 'but the threat did increase sexual arousal. And when you go to bed with someone for the first time, in theory it ought not to succeed. But at a time like that you think of only one thing, and in most cases it works out OK.'

Years ago, in an interview entitled 'Good conversation and a sex film deal with erection problems', a now retired professor of sexology, Koos Slob (1940), gave his urology-unfriendly view: 'Modern diagnostic techniques are so sensitive that if you or I go to the urologist some abnormality or other will always be found. But whether it will actually cause any problems is highly doubtful.' After which the interviewer remarks that Slob never gives his car a 'major service', but only has essentials like tyres and brakes checked . . .

Not only in this interview but also in his inaugural lecture Slob emphasized his view that in most men with erection problems the cause is psychological. All in the mind, as it were! His nuanced view, however, made him sometimes see virtue in a 'minor' urological service. It has long since ceased to be the case that urologists are wary of directly associating the genitalia with sex and eroticism. There is increasing interest in the influence of the psyche – call it the brain – on individual organs. Typical examples of this are the development of neurocardiology and neurourology.

Slob's inaugural lecture opens in elegantly epigrammatic fashion:

> The softness of our penis escapes our attention. Yet it's just as well that most men have a limp penis for most of the time. We undervalue our genital softness not only because in a patriarchy so many phallic values are acquired, but also because all of us identify masculine energy and real masculinity with the vitality of a youthful male image. As we grow older the degree of hardness of our penis declines. Frightened as we are of our own mortality, we do not want to see our own genital softness and project it onto women, whom we find weak, and soft and vulnerable – all signs of mortality, all qualities to be looked down on and denied . . . The undervaluation of genital softness and overvaluing of the phallus have made the world a dangerous place for men. The price of that undervaluation is the loss of an essential spiritual energy and strength. It is the energy and strength associated with the 'Via Negativa'.

Of course these epigrams, with their echo of Lord Nelson's blind eye to the telescope, have a seductive ring, but such airy notions cut no ice in daily urological practice, and Slob realizes that only too well. The fact remains that urologists and psychologists tend to think rather differently about things. In his heyday a well-known sexologically orientated professor of psychology characterized urological involvement with erection problems as 'plumbing work'. He was forgetting – and one can hardly hold it against him as a non-doctor – that urologists have the reputation of being the most intelligent of all surgical specialists (in other words: they are very bright plumbers). They earn well too – so is that perhaps the problem?

Almost a hundred years ago behaviourists helped prevent fundamental research into the physical causes of ED from getting off the ground. After all, the problem was virtually always psychologically based. This view led to therapeutic nihilism and gave doctors little encouragement for further research. ('You're not twenty any more'.) Consequently, at the point where the first man walked on the moon, knowledge about erections did not extend beyond the fact that 'cushions' in the erectile tissue compartments in the penis might be able to retain blood.

In the past few decades much ground has been made up, especially since the introduction of Viagra. Scientists from different disciplines seized on the erection, and the same thing happened with male fertility problems. Yet modesty is still in order. Scientific findings reflect only a very small part of everyday reality, which is often so bitter. Writers and poets, major and minor, male and female, undoubtedly give a broader, more human view of reality. Ample evidence proves the truth of that statement. Erection problems and fertility disorders hurt less when writers, poets and philosophers reflect on them. In that way reading comes to resemble a form of mental surgery, in which one's 'suffering' is placed in a broader perspective.

The double flame

One thing is certain: sexuality, including sexual potency, is nature's great engine, and reproduction constitutes the natural basis of our existence – there is no escaping and no denying it. So respect for sexuality, but also respect for the problems of the impotent man is called for. Many people cannot summon up that respect. The hatred for men who are unable to make full use of their genitalia has existed since time immemorial. Obviously little can be done about it, or about erectile dysfunction and infertility, since in many cases problems cannot be solved.

Growing old is often accompanied by an unpleasant physical decline, and that will probably always remain so. But in the twenty-first century we live in a society in which the healthy, vital, young, beautiful and potent body has become the yardstick. In fact the ideal of the body as 'the eternally and efficiently functioning machine' is based on suppression, not only in contemporary technological and information-based culture, but by ourselves, the suppression of the undeniable reality that each of us inhabits a body that is transient, that can break down, that can get ill and one day will die. So for many men it is often a great relief if for a change they can speak freely about feelings of impotence, fear of failure or apparent resignation – not only resignation about impotence but ultimate resignation in the face of death.

Besides the reproductive function of sex, with its help we human beings can reinforce our sense of 'togetherness'. Sexual relations can revitalize us, and can bring relief where there are tensions. It is an excellent form of relaxation and recreation and apart from that it is better than a sleeping pill. Whether we actually experience it like that in practice, is another matter. More than many people think, our sexual experience is linked to an involvement, which may or may not be conscious, with the purpose of our existence; with being satisfied or otherwise with the role we are playing in this world and with the love with which we may or may not know or feel we are connected. More than we think, our sexual behaviour obeys obscure powers of which we are only vaguely, if at all, aware.

The Nobel Prize-winning Mexican poet and essayist Octavio Paz described in *The Double Flame* his view of the relationship between sexuality, reproduction, eroticism and love. The red of the flame stands, he believes, for the primitive instinct of sexuality, which we share with animals. Further inside the flame burns yellow: the play aspect of eroticism, which in every culture gives eroticism a human face. The centre of the flame burns transparent blue: there sexuality and eroticism are purified into the essentially human capacity for love.

According to Paz eroticism can free itself from sexuality. Flames change, they flicker. In this way eroticism diverts sexuality from its evolutionary goal, reproduction. But that change, that separation, is paradoxically at the same time a return. The human couple making love find their way to the sea of sex and are rocked by the endless, gentle waves. There they rediscover the innocence of wild animals. 'Eroticism is a rhythm' concludes Paz, 'one of its chords is separation, the other is return, the journey back to reconciled nature. The erotic beyond is here, and it is this very moment. All women and all men have lived such moments; it is our share of paradise.'

conclusion

That Wraps it Up

In the second century AD the physician Galen wrote: 'The testicles are more important than the heart; the heart serves to keep us alive, the testicles to make us truly alive.' Being 'truly' alive takes its toll. In that respect eunuchs were men without ballast. If one studies the operation of testosterone closely, one has the impression that it is a very cunning invention. The hormone drives one to fight, to be aggressive, and weakens the immune system. It seems as if men are doomed to have to prove how strong they are to women. They have to show in some way that the genetic material in their sperm is good quality. Partly because of that, testosterone leads to useless antlers, tail feathers that are yards long and in men to premature baldness.

The 'noble' parts are in my view 'casual staff'. They must be treated properly or they inevitably down tools. Excessive alcohol consumption, smoking, anabolic steroids, intensive pursuit of sports (marathon runners almost invariably have poor seed and racing cyclists have numb genitals after a long ride), underpants that are too warm, tight jeans, frequent saunas and endless hours in a warm bath are things a man should avoid.

More and more frequently men become alarmed about imagined abnormalities in their genitals. Usually these are innocuous ailments. Even prostate cancer can be included among these in many cases.

Worshipped in ancient religions, then demonized by the Church fathers, secularized by learned anatomists and physiologists like Leonardo da Vinci, Reinier de Graaf and Anthony van Leeuwenhoek, and then for a while subjected to psychoanalysis by Sigmund Freud: the 'noble parts' have been through quite a lot. After being praised to the skies by psychologists, abused by feminists and shamelessly exploited in pop culture, in the twenty-first century they are in danger of becoming totally medicalized. The erection and reproductive industries are developing apace. The 'noble' parts must not fail, the repeated resurrection of the flesh must continue to manifest itself. In cases where the reproductive mechanism fails there is support, as if it were perfectly normal. Darwin is defied, the human race can only become weaker, with debilitating ailments, en route for the end, the apocalypse.

Human suffering, bell-ringing, testicles, sperm, testosterone and testament are woven by poet Frederik Lucien de Laere into a harmonious, apocalyptic apotheosis entitled 'Creation':

> It has been made, the testament.
> The final testicle's produced the final seed
> and testosterone has sired a bald head.
>
> After each big bang
> millions of cells were
> hurled into space
> (cell shock, good God!)
> They fought their way
> through the expansiveness
> in search of Columbus's egg.
>
> The pure globe shapes
> once housed the origin
> till the gong
> boomed so loud
> that it all blew up
> and the dust of stars
> spread across the heath,
> the far and wide of the woman.
> Now the emission has stopped
> it hangs there quietly, its peal of bells
> laid down by the music of the spheres.

Bibliography

INTRODUCTION

Belt, E., 'Leonardo the Florentine', *Investigative Urology*, III (1965), I
Graaf, R. de, *Virorum organis inservientibus, de clysteribus et usu siphonis in anatomia* (Rotterdam, 1668)

I THE TESTICLES AND THE SCROTUM

Cobb, M., *The Egg and Sperm Race: The Seventeenth-Century Scientists Who Unravelled the Secrets of Sex, Life and Growth* (London, 2007)
Colledge, E., *Reynard the Fox and Other Medieval Netherlands Secular Literature* (Leiden, London and New York, 1967)
Havelock Ellis, H., *Studies in the Psychology of Sex*, 8 vols (New York, 1936)
Gould, G. M. and W. L. Pyle, *Anomalies and Curiosities of Medicine* (New York, 1956)
Jong, E., *Fear of Flying* (London, 1974)
Hunter, J., *Essays and Observations* 2 vols (London, 1861), p. 189
Mitsya, H., J. Asai, K. Suyama, T. Ushida and K. Hosoe, 'Application of x-ray cinematography in urology. 1. Mechanism of ejaculation', *Journal of Urology*, LXXXIII (1960), 86–92
Rolnick, D., S. Kawanode and P. Szanto, 'Anatomical incidence of testicular appendages', *Journal of Urology*, C (1969), 755–6
Sands, D. B., ed., *The History of Reynard the Fox: Translated by William Caxton in 1481* (Cambridge, MA, and London, 1960)
Williams, G., *Sexual Language and Imagery in Shakespearean and Stuart Literature*, 3 vols (London and Atlantic Highlands, NJ, 1996)

2 THE PENIS

Belt, E., 'Leonardo the Florentine', *Investigative Urology*, III (1965), I
Cobb, M., *The Egg and Sperm Race: The Seventeenth-Century Scientists Who Unravelled the Secrets of Sex, Life and Growth* (London, 2007)
Courtade, D., *Notions practiques d'électrothérapie appliqué à l'urologie* (Paris, 1921)

Dekkers, M., *Dearest Pet: On Bestiality*, trans. P. Vincent (London and New York, 1994)

Eckhardt, C., 'Untersuchungen über die Erektion des Penis beim Hund', *Beitragen Anatomie und Physiologie*, III (1863), 123

Feldman, K. W. and D. W. Smith, 'Fetal phallic growth and penile standards for new born male infants', *Journal of Pediatrics*, LXXXVI (1975), 395

Fisher, W., N. Branscombe and C. Lemery, 'The bigger the better? Arousal and attributional responses to erotic stimuli that depict different size penises', *Journal of Sex Research*, XIX (1983), 377

de Graaf, R., *Virorum organis inservientibus, de clysteribus et usu siphonis in anatomia* (Rotterdam, 1668)

Griffin, G., *Penis Enlargement Methods – Fact & Phallusy*, 9th edn (Palm Springs, CA, 1996)

Hawley, R. M. and J. H. Owens, 'Koro: its presentation in an elderly male', *International Journal of Geriatric Psychiatry*, III (1988), 69–72

Kamvisseli, E., *F/32* (Boulder, CO, Normal, IL, and Brooklyn, NY, 1990)

Lawrence, D. H., *Lady Chatterley's Lover* (Florence, 1928)

Loeb, H., 'Harnröhren und Tripperspritzen', *Münchener Medizinische Wochenschrift*, XLVI (1899), 10–19

Malnick, C., J. A. Flaherty and T. Jobe, 'Koro: how culturally specific?', *International Journal of Social Psychiatry*, XXXI (1985), 67

McCarthy, B., *Sexual Awareness: A Practical Approach* (San Francisco, CA, 1975)

Moravia, A., *The Two of Us*, trans. A. Davidson (London, 1972)

Sheikh Nefzawi, *The Perfumed Garden*, trans. Sir R. F. Burton (London, 1965)

Pluijm, C. van der, 'Piemels. Over geslachtsdelen', *Gay Krant* (September 1994)

Payne Knight, R. and T. Wright, *A History of Phallic Worship* (New York, 1992)

Piesol, S. A., *Human Anatomy* (Philadelphia, PA, 1907)

Ponce de León, S. A., F. Algaba and J. Salvador, 'Cutaneous horn of glans penis', *British Journal of Urology*, LXXIV (1994), 257

Sagan, F., *A Certain Smile* (London, 1956)

Scott, G.R., *Phallic Worship* (Westport, CT, 1956)

Siminosky, K. and J. Bain, 'The relationships among height, penile length and foot size', *Annals of Sex Research*, 6 (1993), 231–5

Thomas, P., *Kama Kalpa or The Hindu Road to Love* (Bombay, 1959)

Vroon, P., A. van Amerongen and H. Vries, *Smell: The Secret Seducer*, trans. Paul Vincent (New York, 1997)

Wen-Shing Tseng, Mo Kan-Ming, Jing Hsu, Li Li Shuen, Ou Li-Wah, Chen Guo-Qian and Jiang Da-Wei, 'A sociocultural study of koro epidemics in Guangdong, China', *American Journal of Psychiatry*, CXLV (1988), 15–38

X, Dr Jacobus, *Untrodden Fields of Anthropology* (Paris, 1898)

Zilbergeld, B., *Men and Sex: A Guide to Self-Fulfilment* (London, 1980)

3 THE PROSTATE AND SEMINAL GLANDS

Boyard, A., *Intoxicated by My Illness and Other Writings on Life and Death* (New York, 1992)

Ceronetti, G., *The Silence of the Body* (New York, 1994)

Malcolm, N., *Ludwig Wittgenstein: A Memoir* (New York, 1958)

Monk, R., *Ludwig Wittgenstein: The Duty of Genius* (London, 1990)

Zaviacic, M., *The Human Female Prostate* (Bratislava, 1999)

4 TESTOSTERONE AND SPERM

Buhl, W., *Eros mit grauen Schläfen* (Rüschlikon, 1961)

Bulgakov, M., *Heart of a Dog*, trans. M. Ginsburg (New York, 1987)

Cobb, M., *The Egg and Sperm Race: The Seventeenth-Century Scientists Who Unravelled the Secrets of Sex, Life and Growth* (London, 2007)

Courtade, D., *Notions practiques d'électrothérapie appliqué à l'urologie* (Paris, 1921)

Dekkers, M., *Dearest Pet: On Bestiality*, trans. P. Vincent (London and New York, 1994)

Dufour, P., and F. Helbing, *Geschiedenis der Sexueele Zeden* (Zalt-Bomusel, 1910)

Kruif, P. de, *The Male Hormone* (New York, 1945)

Kundera, M., *Farewell Waltz*, trans. A. Asher (London, 1998)

Lowsley, O. S. and E. A. Rueda, 'Further experience with an operation for the cure of certain types of impotence', *Journal of the International College of Surgeons*, xix (1953), 69

Lydston, G. F., 'The surgical treatment of impotence', *American Journal of Clinical Medicine*, xv (1908), 1571

Margulis, L. and D. Sagon, *Origins of Sex: Three Billion Years of Genetic Recombination* (New Haven, CT, 1986)

Partington, A., *The Oxford Library of Words and Phrases. 1 Quotations* (Oxford, 1993)

Shakespeare, W., *The Winter's Tale*, in *The Complete Works of William Shakespeare*, ed. W. J. Craig (London, 1990)

Steinach, E. and J. Loebel, *Sex and Life* (London, 1939)

Voronoff, S., *Testicular Grafting from Ape to Man*, trans. T. Merrill (London, 1930)

Waldinger, M. D., P. Quinn, M. Dilleen, R. Mundayat, D. H. Schweitzer and M. Boolell, 'A multinational population survey on Intravaginal Ejaculation Latency Time', *Journal of Sexual Medicine*, ii (2002), 492–7

Walton, A.H., 'The story of testosterone and rejuvenation', in *Aphrodisiacs: from Legend to Prescription* (Westport, CT, 1958)

5 CASTRATION

Aucoin, M. W. and R. J. Wasserzug, 'The sexuality and social performance of androgen-deprived (castrated) men throughout history: implications for modern day cancer patients', *Social Science and Medicine*, 63 (2006), 3162–73

Barbier, P., *The World of the Castrati: The History of an Extraordinary Operatic Phenomenon* (London, 1996)

Darmon, P., *Damning the Innocent* (London, 1986)

Engelstein, L., *Castration and the Heavenly Kingdom* (New York, 1999)

Finer, S., *The History of Government from the Earliest Times* (Oxford, 1999)

Friedman, D., *A Mind of its Own* (New York, 2001)

Koch, W., *Über die Russisch-Rumänische Kastratensekte der Skopzen* (Jena, 1921)

Moreschi, A., *Rossini's Petite Messe Solonelle*, EMI CD (1994) France 5 55054 2; *The Last Castrato (The Vatican Recordings)*, Pearl OPAL CD 9823

Newman, R. J., *The Silence of Men* (Fort Lee, NJ, 2005)

Ranke-Heinemann, U., *Eunuchs for the Kingdom of Heaven: Women, Sexuality, and the Catholic Church*, trans. P. Heinegg (New York, 1991)

Sushruta Samhita, An English Translation Based on the Original Sanskrit Text (Varanasi, 1963)

Taylor, G., *Castration: An Abbreviated History of Western Manhood* (New York, 2000)

6 AILMENTS OF THE SCROTUM

Barten, E., *Experimental Homologous Testis Transplantation* (Amsterdam, 1997)

Gould, G. M. and W. L. Pyle, *Anomalies and Curiosities of Medicine* (New York, 1956)

Hakami, M. and S. H. Mosavy, 'Triorchidism with normal spermatogenesis: an unusual case for failure of vasectomy', *British Journal of Surgery*, LXII (1975), 633–6

Vargas Llosa, M., *The Feast of the Goat*, trans. E. Grossman (London, 2001)

Voorhoeve, B., *Door de pijngrens* (Utrecht, 2000) adapted from L. Armstrong with S. Jenkins, *It's Not About the Bike: My Journey Back to Life* (London, 2000)

7 AILMENTS OF THE PENIS

Beheri, G. E., 'Surgical treatment of impotence', *Plastic and Reconstructive Surgery*, XXXVIII (1960), 92

Bernant, G., 'Sexual behaviour: hard time with the Coolidge effect', in *Psychological Research: The Inside Story*, ed. M. H. Siegel and H. P. Ziegler (New York, 1976)

Bett, W. R., 'The os penis in man and beast', *Proceedings of the Royal Society of Medicine*, XLIV (1951), 433

Bogoras, N. A., 'Über die volle plastische Wiederherstellung eines zum Koïtus fähigen Penis', *Zentralblatt Chirurgie*, XXII (1936), 1271

Botton, A. de, *The Consolations of Philosophy* (London, 2000)

Chang, J., *The Tao of Love and Sex: The Ancient Chinese Way to Ecstasy* (London, 1991)

Culicchia, G., 'Fuori programma', in *Papergang Under 25 vol. III* (Massa, 1990)

Darmon, P., *Le tribunal de l'impuissance* (Paris, 1979)

Havelock Ellis, H., *Studies in the Psychology of Sex*, 8 vols (New York, 1936)

Erikson, C. J. P., T. Fukunaga and R. Lindman, 'Sex hormone response to alcohol', *Nature* (30 June 1974), 711

Fiebag, J. and P. Fiebag, *Die Ewigkeits-Maschine* (Munich, 1998)

Fontana, P., 'Il taccuino', in *Bersagli* (Venice, 1993)

Goethe, J. W. von, *Erotic Poems*, trans. D. Luke (Oxford, 1997)

Gollaher, D. L., *Circumcision – A History of the World's Most Controversial Surgery* (New York, 2000)

Brothers Grimm, *The Complete Fairy Tales* (Ware, 2009)

Gutheil, E. A., *The Autobiography of Wilhelm Stekel* (New York, 1950)

Raphael, B. and A. Nash, 'In bed with Elvis', *Playboy* (November 2005)

Irving, J., *The World According to Garp* (London, 1978)

Kama Sutra of Vatsyayana, Translated from the Sanskrit (London, 1883)

Kinsey, A. C., W. B. Pomeroy and C. E. Martin, *Sexual Behaviour in the Male* (Philadelphia, PA, 1948)

Kundera, M., *Farewell Waltz*, trans. A. Asher (London, 1998)

Lange, J., *Die Folgen der Entmannung Erwachsener* (Leipzig, 1934)

Lawrence, D. H., *Lady Chatterley's Lover* (Florence, 1928)

Lowsley, O. S. and E. A. Rueda, 'Further experience with an operation for the cure of certain types of impotence', *Journal of the International College of Surgeons*, XIX (1953), 69

Lydston, G. F., 'The surgical treatment of impotence', *American Journal of Clinical Medicine*, XV (1908), 1571

de Maupassant, G., 'Le moyen de Roger and Rouille', *Contes et Nouvelles* (Paris, 1980)

Miller, H., *Tropic of Cancer* (Paris, 1934)

Moll, A., *Handbuch der Sexualwissenschaften* (Leipzig, 1912)

Parker, W. H., *Priapea: Poems for a Phallic God* (London, 1988)

Parona, D., 'Imperfetta erezione del pene per varicosità della vena dorsale: osservazione', *Giornale Italiano delle Malattie Veneree e della Pelle*, XIV (1873), 7

Pavese, C., *The Business of Living: Diaries 1935–1950*, trans. A. E. Murch (with J. Molli) (New Brunswick, NJ, and London, 2009)

Paz, O., *The Double Flame: Love and Eroticism*, trans. H. Lane (San Diego, CA, New York and London, 1995)

Robbins, H., *The Betsy* (London, 1971)

Roubaud, J., *Traité de l'impuissance* (Paris, 1876)

Rousseau, J. J., *Confessions*, trans. J. M. Cohen (London, 1953)

Russell, G. L., 'Impotence treated by mechanotherapy', *Proceedings of the Royal Society of Medicine*, LIX (1959), 872

Servadio, G., *The Story of R*, trans. A. Mostyn-Owen (London, Sydney and Auckland, 1994)

Shakespeare, W., *Macbeth*, in *The Complete Works of William Shakespeare*, ed. W. J. Craig (London, 1990)

Sigerist, H. E., 'Impotence as result of witchcraft', in *Essays in Biology* (Berkeley, CA, 1943)

Sprenger, J. and H. Institoris, *Malleus Maleficarum* (New York, 1971)

Stekel, W., *Die Impotenz des Mannes* (Berlin and Vienna, 1920)

Sushruta Samhita, An English Translation Based on the Original Sanskrit Text (Varanasi, 1963)

Tolstoy, L., *Anna Karenina*, trans. R. Edmonds (Harmondsworth, 1954)

Unsfeld, S., *Das Tagebuch Goethes und Rilkes Sieben Gedichte* (Frankfurt am Main, 1978)

Vecki, V. G., *The Pathology and Treatment of Sexual Impotence: From the Author's Second German Edition, Revised and Rewritten* (Philadelphia, PA, 1899)

Virag, R., 'Intracavernous injection of papaverine for erectile failure', *Lancet*, 2 (1982), 938

Weyer, J., *De Praestigiis Daemonum*, Libris IV, Capitum XX; also *On Witchcraft: an Abridged Translation of Johann Weyer's* De Praestigiis Daemonum, trans. J. Shea (Asheville, NC, 1998)

Zhisui Li, *The Private Life of Chairman Mao*, trans. A. F. Thurston (London, 1994)

Zeegers, W., *De zonnige zijde van seks; de nawerking van positief beleefde sexualiteit* (Leiden, 1994)

Zilbergeld, B., *Men and Sex: A Guide to Sexual Fulfilment* (London, 1980)

8 VOLUNTARY AND INVOLUNTARY STERILITY

Bardenheuer, B., 'Mitteilungen aus dem Kölner Bürgerhospital', *Zentralblatt Chirurgie*, XV (1888), 367

Ranke-Heinemann, U., *Eunuchs for the Kingdom of Heaven: Women, Sexuality, and the Catholic Church*, trans. P. Heinegg (New York, 1991)

Spath, F., 'Über Samenleiter-Sperroperationen. Ein Beitrag zur Kentniss der Sterilisierungsoperationen und zur Frage der Rückoperationen', *Archiv der Klinischen Chirurgie*, CLXXVIII (1934), 737

9 SPILLING ONE'S SEED

Bockting, W. O. and E. Coleman, *Masturbation as a Means of Achieving Sexual Health* (New York, 2002)

Chang, J., *The Tao of Love and Sex: The Ancient Chinese Way to Ecstasy* (London, 1991)

von Goethe, J. W., *Truth and Fiction*, trans. J. Oxenford, available at www.gutenberg.org/etext/5733, accessed 25 June 2009

Gogol, N. V., *Diary of a Madman and Other Stories*, trans. R. Wilks (Harmondsworth, 1972)

Hammond, W. A., *Sexual Impotence in the Male and Female* (Detroit, MI, 1887, repr. New York, 1974)

Havelock Ellis, H., *Studies in the Psychology of Sex*, 8 vols (New York, 1936)

Hite, S., *The Hite Report on Male Sexuality* (New York, 1981)

Kinsey, A. C., W. B. Pomeroy and C. E. Martin, *Sexual Behaviour in the Male* (Philadelphia, PA, 1948)

Laqueur, T. W., *Solitary Sex: A Social History of Masturbation* (Cambridge, MA, 2003)

Mountjoy, P. T., 'Some early attempts to modify penile erection in horse and human: an historical analysis', *Psychological Record*, XXIV (1974), 291–308

Roth, P., *Portnoy's Complaint* (London, 1969)

Rousseau, J. J., *Confessions*, trans. J. M. Cohen (London, 1953)

Stengers, J. and A. Van Neck, *Masturbation: The History of a Great Terror*, trans. K. Hoffmann (New York, 2001)

Tissot, S. A., *Traité de l'Onanisme: Dissertation sur les Maladies produites par la Masturbation* (Lausanne, 1764)

Toole, J. K., *A Confederacy of Dunces* (Harmondsworth, 1981)

10 WOMEN

Cats, J., *Alle de wercken van den Heere Jacob Cats* (Amsterdam and The Hague, 1726), II, 166a

Janssen, E., 'Provoking penile responses', dissertation, University of Amsterdam, Faculty of Psychology, 1995

Jong, E., *Fear of Flying* (London, 1974)

Kamvisseli, E., *F/32* (Boulder, CO, Normal, IL, and Brooklyn, NY, 1990)

Venette, N., *Conjugal Love, or the Pleasure of the Marriage Bed* (London, 1984)

11 EROTICISM

Bataille, G., *Visions of Excess: Selected Writings, 1927–1939*, trans. A. Stoekl (Minneapolis, MN, 1985)

——, *The Story of the Eye*, trans. J. Neugroschel (London, 1979)

Havelock Ellis, H., *Studies in the Psychology of Sex*, 8 vols (New York, 1936)

Janssen, E., 'Provoking penile responses', dissertation, University of Amsterdam, Faculty of Psychology, 1995

Kinsey, A. C., W. B. Pomeroy and C. E. Martin, *Sexual Behaviour in the Male* (Philadelphia, PA, 1948)

MacKenzie, B. and E. MacKenzie, *It's Not All in Your Head* (New York, 1988)

Masters, W. H. and V. E. Johnson, *Human Sexual Inadequacy* (London, 1970)

Paz, O., *The Double Flame: Love and Eroticism*, trans. Helen Lane (San Diego, CA, New York and London, 1995)

Acknowledgements

Working in a university means being prepared to collaborate with other disciplines. Sexology is very well suited to this. In it you find general practitioners, gynaecologists, urologists, psychotherapists, psychologists, biologists, social workers, historians and occasionally 'oddballs'. Recently I had the privilege of working with a jaw surgeon who was doing a doctorate on the 'sleep apnoea syndrome' and had brought sex into it.

Sexologists based in the north of the Netherlands have close ties and encourage each other wherever possible, for example by writing popular-scientific books or chapters in academic volumes. On this occasion I should like to mention Jelto Drenth and Willibrord Weijmar Schultz by name.

Without Ab Oost, a bibliophile from Deventer, I would never have been able to write my books and articles. He has been responsible to a considerable degree for my acquiring a very large collection of antiquarian books on male impotence.

Koos Meuzelaar, a thoracic surgeon but also a very well-read clergyman's son, lent me relevant medical-historical works, of which I have made extensive use.

Since my appointment (1983) at the Groningen University Medical Centre – according to an Italian journal the most beautiful hospital building in Europe – Douwe Buiter has always been prepared to provide illustrations free of charge, for which I am most grateful. He is one of the many unassuming, dedicated members of staff in our hospital.

I also want to thank the Members of the Boards of the Professor Piet Boer Foundation for Urology and the Foundation for the Production and Translation of Dutch Literature, who made the translation of this book into English possible. Finally, my editor Peter Claessens put me on the right track. I was in danger of opting for the 'narrow' path, but he led me towards the 'broad' highway, on which the phallus and the testicle remained connected. 'A man – not even you – should not put asunder what the Creator has joined together inextricably for all eternity', was his judgement.

Index